THE VARICOSITY HANDBOOK

WHAT EVERY PATIENT SHOULD KNOW

DR. MOHAMMAD E. BARBATI

Copyright © 2023 by Dr. Mohammad E. Barbati

All rights reserved.

No part of this book may be reproduced in any form or by any electronic or mechanical means, including information storage and retrieval systems, without written permission from the author, except for the use of brief quotations in a book review.

PART ONE
INTRODUCTION TO VARICOSITY

Varicosity, commonly known as varicose veins, is a prevalent vascular disorder that affects millions of people worldwide. This condition is characterized by the presence of enlarged, twisted, and often visible veins, primarily occurring in the legs and feet. While many consider varicose veins to be merely a cosmetic concern, they can significantly impact an individual's quality of life and potentially lead to more serious health complications if left untreated.

DEFINITION AND OVERVIEW

Varicosity refers to the abnormal dilation and elongation of veins, typically in the lower extremities. These affected veins become enlarged, twisted, and protrude beneath the surface of the skin, often appearing as rope-like or bulging blue or purple lines.

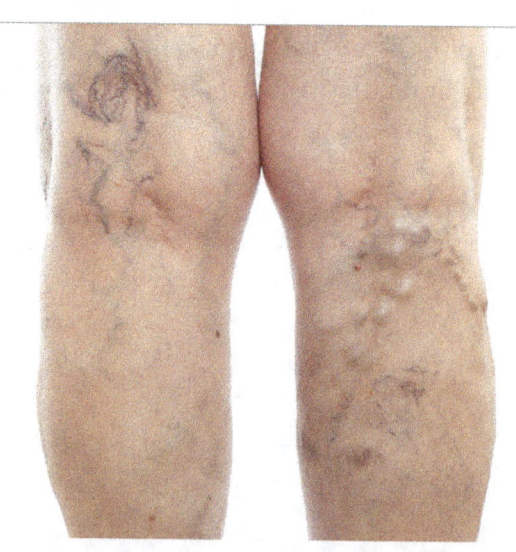

The condition primarily affects the superficial veins, which are closer to the skin's surface, rather than the deep veins responsible for the majority of blood flow back to the heart.

The primary cause of varicosity lies in the malfunctioning of venous valves. Veins contain small, one-way valves that open to allow blood to flow towards the heart and close to prevent backward flow. When these valves become weak or damaged, they fail to close properly, allowing blood to flow backward and pool in the veins. This pooling of blood leads to increased pressure within the veins, causing them to dilate and become varicose.

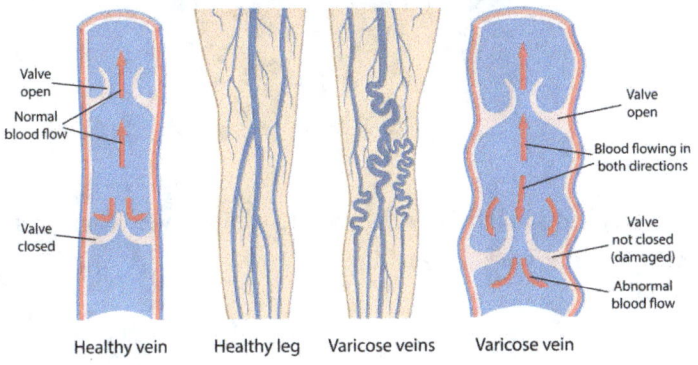

Varicosity is not limited to a single vein type or location. While most commonly observed in the legs, particularly in the calves and thighs, varicose veins can occur in various parts of the body. Some common types of varicosities include:

Saphenous vein varicosities: Affecting the long superficial veins running along the inner thigh and leg

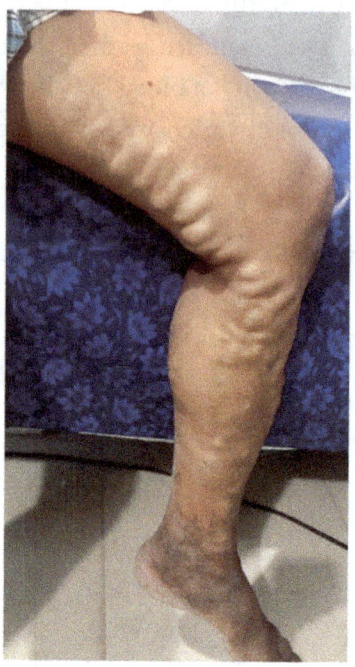

Reticular varicosities: Smaller, dilated veins that often appear as a network of blue lines

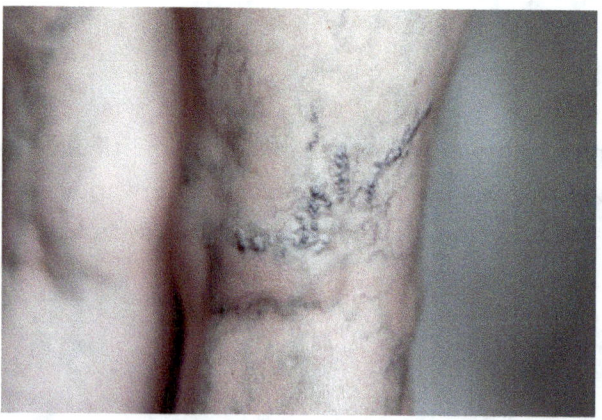

Spider veins: Tiny, thread-like veins visible on the skin's surface, often appearing in a spider web pattern

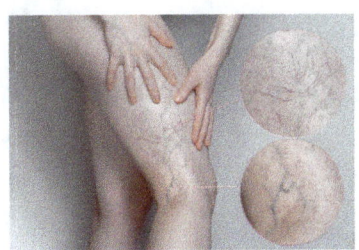

It's important to note that varicosity is not just a cosmetic issue. While the visible appearance of varicose veins can cause distress and self-consciousness, the condition can also lead to various symptoms and potential complications. These may include:

- Aching or heavy legs
- Swelling in the ankles and feet
- Itching or burning sensation around the affected veins
- Skin changes, such as discoloration or hardening
- Increased risk of blood clots
- Development of venous ulcers in severe cases

Understanding the underlying causes and potential consequences of varicosity is crucial for both patients and healthcare providers in managing this condition effectively.

PREVALENCE AND IMPACT ON QUALITY OF LIFE

Varicosity is a widespread condition that affects a significant portion of the global population. While exact prevalence rates vary depending on the study and population examined, it is estimated that approximately 20-25% of adults worldwide are affected by varicose veins. The prevalence increases with age, with up to 50% of individuals over the age of 50 experiencing some form of varicosity.

Several factors contribute to the high prevalence of varicosity:

Age: As individuals grow older, the risk of developing varicose veins increases due to natural wear and tear on vein valves.

Gender: Women are more likely to develop varicose veins than men, with some studies suggesting that women are up to twice as likely to be affected.

Genetics: Family history plays a significant role, with individuals having a parent with varicose veins being more likely to develop the condition.

Lifestyle factors: Prolonged standing or sitting, obesity, and lack of physical activity can contribute to the development of varicose veins.

Pregnancy: Hormonal changes and increased blood volume during pregnancy can increase the risk of varicosity.

The impact of varicosity on an individual's quality of life can be substantial and multifaceted. While some people may experience minimal symptoms, others may face significant physical discomfort and emotional distress. The effects of varicosity on quality of life can be categorized into several areas:

Physical Discomfort: Many individuals with varicose veins experience pain, aching, heaviness, and fatigue in their legs. This discomfort can limit mobility and interfere with daily activities, potentially leading to a more sedentary lifestyle.

Aesthetic Concerns: The visible appearance of varicose veins can cause self-consciousness and negatively impact body image. This may lead to changes in clothing choices and avoidance of activities that expose the legs.

Emotional Well-being: The combination of physical discomfort and aesthetic concerns can contribute to emotional distress, including anxiety and depression in some cases.

Sleep Disturbances: Leg pain and restlessness associated with varicosity can interfere with sleep quality, leading to fatigue and decreased daytime productivity.

Work and Social Life: Severe symptoms may impact an individual's ability to perform certain job functions, particularly those requiring prolonged standing. Social activities may also be limited due to discomfort or embarrassment.

Financial Burden: The costs associated with managing varicosity, including medical treatments and compression garments, can place a financial strain on individuals and healthcare systems.

Potential Complications: The risk of developing more serious complications, such as venous ulcers or deep vein thrombosis, can cause anxiety and require ongoing medical attention.

It's important to recognize that the impact of varicosity on quality of life can vary greatly between individuals. While some may experience minimal effects, others may find the condition significantly impairs their daily functioning and overall well-being. This variability underscores the importance of individualized assessment and treatment approaches in managing varicosity.

As our understanding of varicosity continues to evolve, so do the treatment options and management strategies available to those affected by this condition. By recognizing the prevalence and potential impact of varicosity, healthcare providers and patients can work together to develop effective treatment plans that address both the physical symptoms and quality of life concerns associated with varicose veins.

In the following chapters, we will delve deeper into the anatomy of veins, the underlying causes of varicosity, risk factors, diagnostic methods, and the wide range of treatment options available. By gaining a comprehensive understanding of varicosity, readers will be better equipped to make informed decisions about their vein health and explore the most appropriate management strategies for their individual needs.

PART TWO
THE CIRCULATORY SYSTEM: A BRIEF OVERVIEW

The circulatory system, also known as the cardiovascular system, is a complex network of organs and blood vessels that plays a crucial role in maintaining the body's homeostasis. Its primary function is to transport blood throughout the body, delivering oxygen and nutrients to tissues while removing waste products and carbon dioxide.

The main components of the circulatory system include:
    The heart: A muscular organ that acts as a pump, driving blood through the blood vessels.
    Blood vessels: A network of tubes that carry blood throughout the body, including arteries, veins, and capillaries.
    Blood: The fluid that circulates through the blood vessels, carrying oxygen, nutrients, hormones, and waste products.

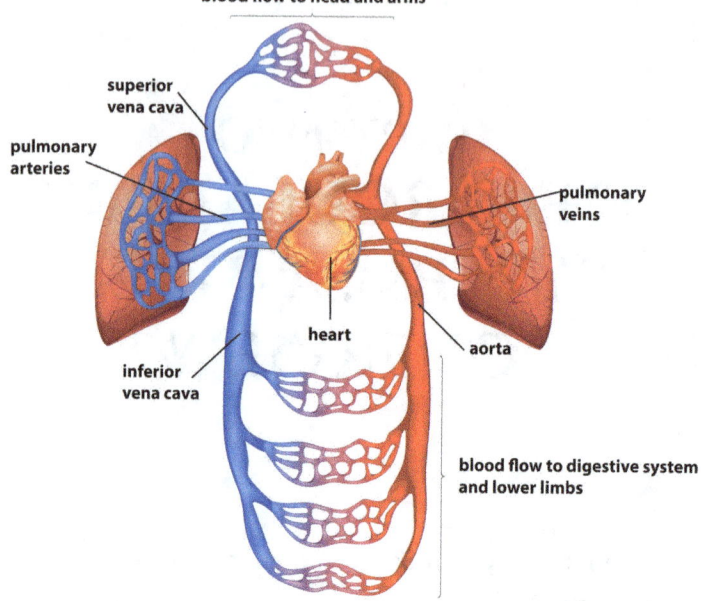

The circulatory system operates in two main circuits:

a) Pulmonary circulation: This circuit involves the movement of blood between the heart and lungs. Deoxygenated blood from the body is pumped to the lungs, where it picks up oxygen and releases carbon dioxide.

b) Systemic circulation: This circuit involves the movement of blood between the heart and the rest of the body. Oxygenated blood from the lungs is pumped to various tissues and organs, delivering oxygen and nutrients while collecting waste products.

DOUBLE CIRCULATION

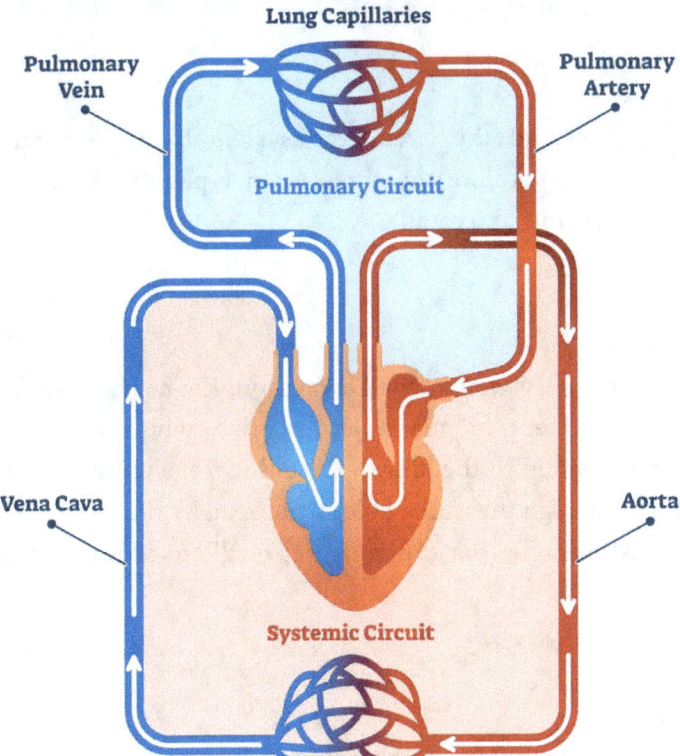

ARTERIES, VEINS, AND CAPILLARIES

To understand the circulatory system in more detail, it's essential to explore the three main types of blood vessels: arteries, veins, and capillaries.

Arteries:

Carry oxygenated blood away from the heart to the body's tissues (except in pulmonary arteries, which carry deoxygenated blood to the lungs). Have thick, elastic walls to withstand the high pressure of blood pumped by the heart. Contain smooth muscle that can constrict or dilate to regulate blood flow.

Veins:

Carry deoxygenated blood from the body's tissues back to the heart (except in pulmonary veins, which carry oxygenated blood from the lungs to the heart). Have thinner walls compared to arteries, as they experience lower blood pressure.

Contain valves to prevent the backflow of blood, especially important in the legs where blood must flow against gravity.

Capillaries:

The smallest blood vessels, connecting arteries and veins.

Have very thin walls (often just one cell thick) to allow for the exchange of gases, nutrients, and waste products between blood and surrounding tissues. Form extensive networks within organs and tissues to maximize the surface area for exchange.

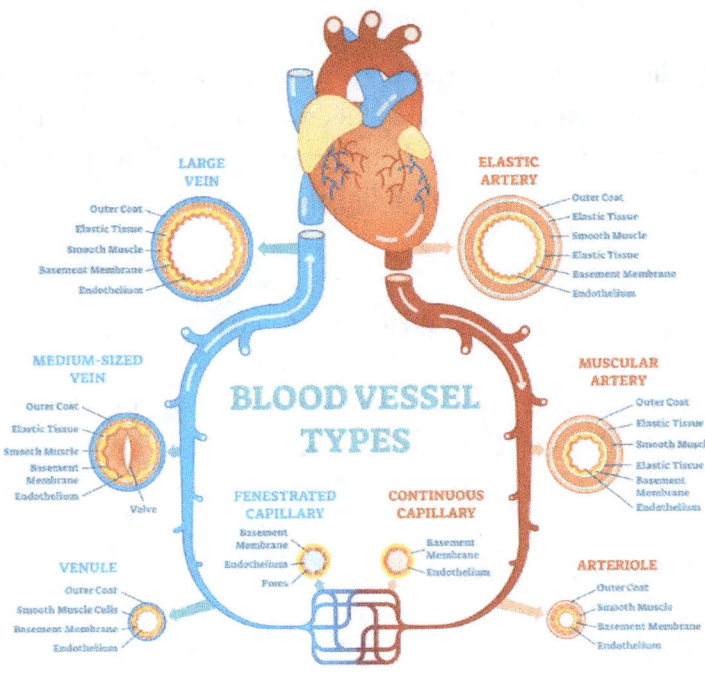

THE ROLE OF VEINS IN BLOOD CIRCULATION

Veins play a crucial role in the circulatory system, particularly in returning deoxygenated blood from the body's tissues back to the heart. Understanding the structure and function of veins is essential for comprehending their role in blood circulation.

Structure of Veins

As mentioned in before, veins have a unique structure that allows them to function effectively:

Three main layers:
a) Tunica Intima: The innermost layer, composed of a thin endothelium that provides a smooth surface for blood flow. This layer also contains valves.
b) Tunica Media: The middle layer, primarily composed of smooth muscle cells and elastic fibers. This layer helps regulate blood flow and allows veins to expand and contract as needed.

c) Tunica Adventitia: The outermost layer, consisting of connective tissue and elastic fibers. It provides structural support to the vein and helps maintain its shape.

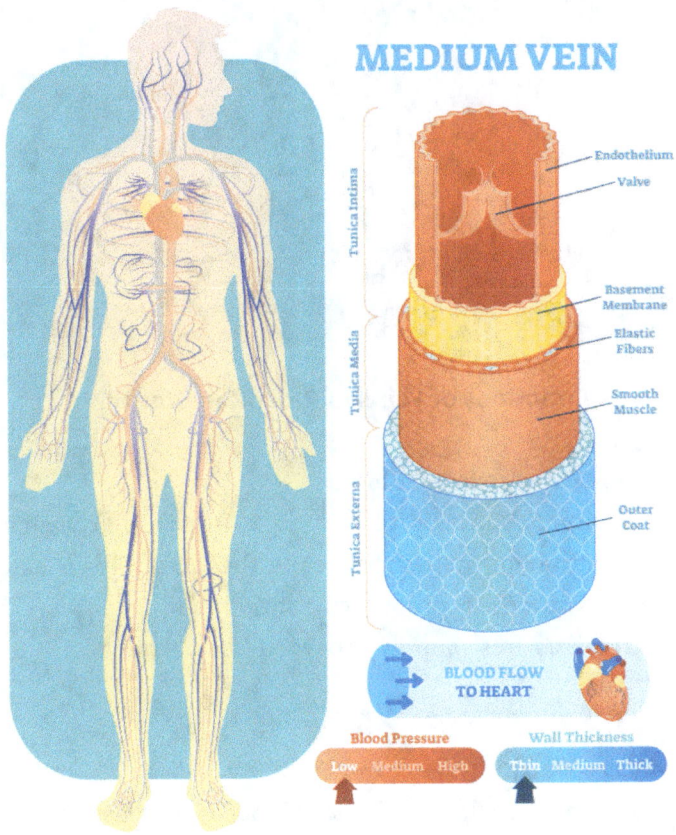

Venous Valves: These are small, flap-like structures found within the lumen of veins. They play a crucial role in maintaining the unidirectional flow of blood towards the heart, preventing backflow or reflux.

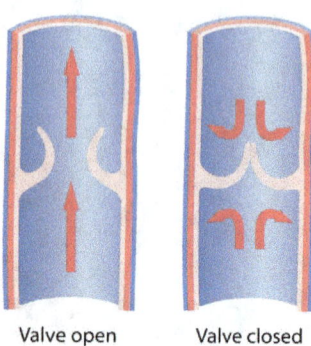

Vein blood circulation

Valve open Valve closed

Functions of Veins in Blood Circulation

Return of Deoxygenated Blood:
The primary function of veins is to return deoxygenated blood from the body's tissues back to the heart. This is essential for maintaining proper circulation and ensuring that tissues receive a fresh supply of oxygen and nutrients.

Blood Reservoir:
Veins can hold a large volume of blood, acting as a reservoir for the circulatory system. This allows the body to adjust blood volume and pressure as needed.

Maintenance of Blood Flow Against Gravity:
Especially in the lower extremities, veins must work against gravity to return blood to the heart. This is achieved through several mechanisms:

a) Venous Valves: These one-way valves prevent the backflow of blood, ensuring that blood moves only towards the heart.

b) Muscle Pump: When surrounding muscles contract, they compress the veins, helping to propel blood upward. This is why walking and other leg movements can help improve circulation.

c) Respiratory Pump: Changes in intrathoracic pressure during breathing can help draw blood towards the heart.

Thermoregulation:

Superficial veins play a role in regulating body temperature. When the body needs to cool down, these veins dilate, bringing more blood close to the skin's surface where heat can be dissipated.

Pressure Regulation:

Veins can constrict or dilate to help regulate blood pressure and blood flow throughout the body.

PART THREE
UNDERSTANDING VARICOSITY

Varicosity, also known as varicose veins, is a common vascular disorder that affects millions of people worldwide. It is characterized by enlarged, twisted veins that are visible beneath the skin's surface, primarily occurring in the legs and feet.

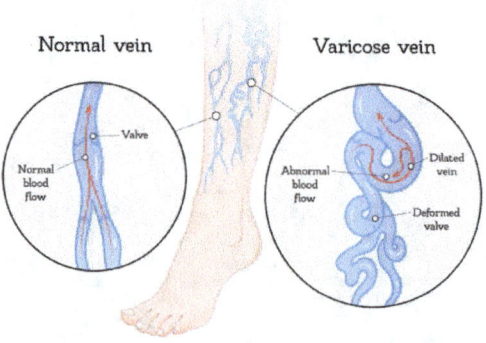

To understand varicosity, it's essential to grasp the following key points:

Definition:

Varicosity refers to a condition where veins become abnormally dilated, elongated, and tortuous. These veins are typically superficial veins, meaning they are closer to the skin's surface.

Primary Affected Areas:
While varicose veins can occur in various parts of the body, they most commonly affect the legs and feet. This is due to the increased pressure these veins experience when working against gravity to return blood to the heart.

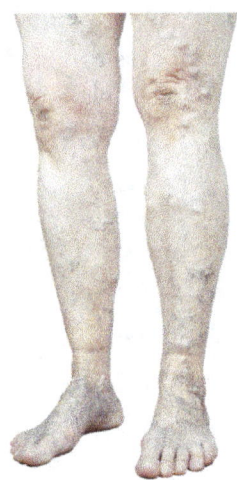

More Than a Cosmetic Issue:
Although varicose veins are often considered a cosmetic concern, they can lead to various complications if left untreated. These may include venous ulcers, blood clots, and chronic venous insufficiency.

Impact on Quality of Life:

Varicosity can significantly impact an individual's quality of life, causing discomfort, pain, and self-consciousness. It may also affect daily activities and lead to more severe health issues if not addressed properly.

Circulatory System Involvement:

To truly understand varicosity, it's crucial to consider its place within the broader circulatory system. Veins are responsible for carrying deoxygenated blood back to the heart, and any disruption in this process can lead to the development of varicose veins.

WHAT CAUSES VARICOSE VEINS

The development of varicose veins is typically attributed to a combination of factors. Understanding these causes is crucial for both prevention and treatment. Here are the main factors that contribute to the formation of varicose veins:

Venous Valve Dysfunction:

The primary cause of varicosity is the malfunctioning of venous valves. Healthy veins contain valves that open to allow blood flow towards the heart and close to prevent backflow. When these valves become weak or damaged, they fail to close properly, allowing blood to flow backward and pool in the veins. This pooling of blood puts additional pressure on the vein walls, causing them to dilate and become varicose.

Increased Venous Pressure:

Factors that increase pressure within the veins can contribute to varicosity. This includes conditions such as obesity, pregnancy, chronic constipation, or tumors that put pressure on the veins. Prolonged standing or sitting can also increase venous pressure, as it hinders the normal flow of blood back to the heart.

Venous Insufficiency:

Chronic venous insufficiency refers to the compromised ability of veins to return blood efficiently to the heart. This condition can lead to increased venous pressure, resulting in the enlargement and twisting of veins.

Age:

As we age, our veins lose elasticity, and the valves may weaken, increasing the risk of varicosity. The natural wear and tear on veins over time can contribute to their dilation and the development of varicose veins.

Genetics:

Family history plays a significant role in the development of varicose veins. Inherited factors can affect the structural integrity of veins and the efficiency of venous valves.

Gender:

Women are more likely to develop varicose veins than men. Hormonal factors, including those related to pregnancy and menopause, contribute to this increased risk.

Pregnancy:

The hormonal changes and increased blood volume during pregnancy can put additional strain on the veins. The growing uterus may also exert pressure on pelvic veins, causing further venous congestion.

Obesity:

Excess weight puts added pressure on the veins, making them more prone to dilation. Obesity also increases the risk of developing other conditions, such as deep vein thrombosis, which can contribute to varicosity.

Lifestyle Factors:

Prolonged standing or sitting, especially in occupations that require these postures for extended periods, can hinder proper blood flow and increase the risk of varicosities. Lack of physical activity can also contribute to poor circulation and increased risk of varicose veins.

Previous Leg Trauma:

A history of leg injuries or trauma, such as fractures or deep vein thrombosis, can damage the veins and impair their function, increasing the risk of developing varicosities.

Inflammation:

Inflammatory processes within the veins can weaken their walls and impair valve function. Conditions such as phlebitis or superficial thrombophlebitis can contribute to the development of varicosities.

Congenital Factors:

In some cases, varicosities may be present at birth or develop early in life due to congenital abnormalities in the structure or function of veins.

Understanding these causes is crucial for developing effective prevention strategies and treatment plans for varicose veins. It's important to note that often, multiple factors contribute to the development of varicosity in an individual.

TYPES OF VARICOSE VEINS

Varicose veins can manifest in various forms, each with its own characteristics and implications. Understanding the different types of varicose veins is essential for proper diagnosis and treatment. Here are the main types of varicose veins:

Trunk Varicose Veins:

These are the most common and noticeable type of varicose veins. They appear as bulging, rope-like veins that are visible beneath the skin's surface.

Trunk varicose veins typically affect the great saphenous vein or the small saphenous vein in the legs. They can cause symptoms such as aching, heaviness, and swelling in the legs.

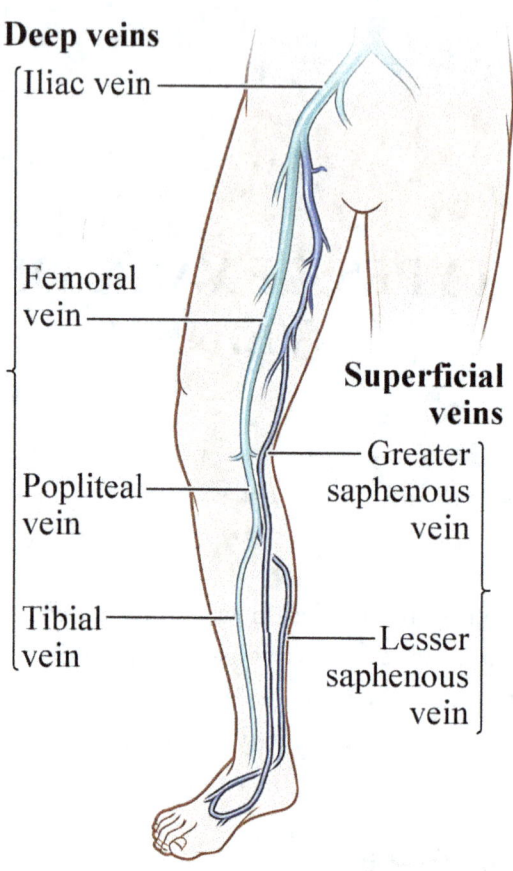

Reticular Veins:

These are smaller, dilated veins that appear as a network of blue or green lines beneath the skin. Reticular veins are often found on the inner thigh or behind the knee. While they may not bulge like trunk varicose veins, they can still cause discomfort and are often associated with spider veins.

Spider Veins (Telangiectasias):

These are the smallest type of varicose veins, appearing as thin, web-like patterns on the skin's surface. Spider veins are typically red, purple, or blue in color. They are most commonly found on the legs but can also appear on the face or other parts of the body. While often considered a cosmetic issue, spider veins can sometimes cause itching or burning sensations.

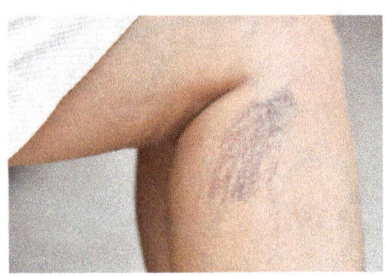

Varicoceles:

These are varicose veins that develop in the scrotum of males. Varicoceles can affect fertility and cause discomfort or a heavy feeling in the scrotum.

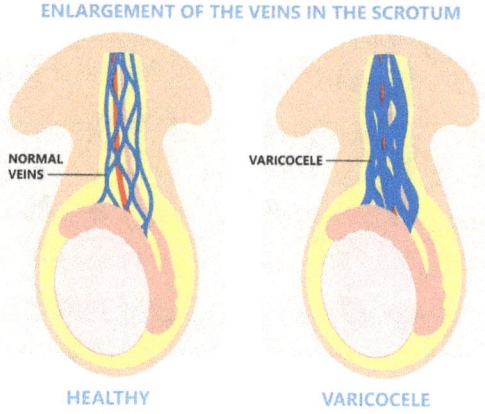

Hemorrhoids:

These are varicose veins that develop in and around the anus and rectum. Hemorrhoids can cause pain, itching, and bleeding during bowel movements.

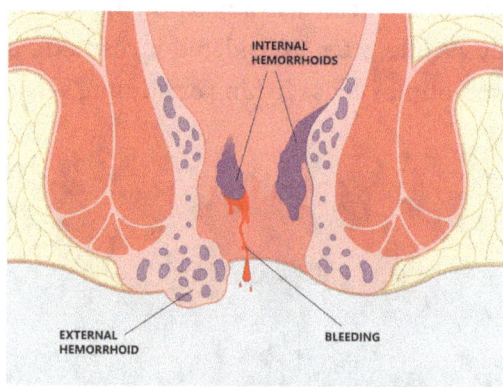

Vulvar Varicosities:

These are varicose veins that develop in the vulva in women. They are often associated with pregnancy and can cause discomfort in the pelvic area.

Corona Phlebectatica:

This refers to a fan-shaped pattern of small, dilated veins on the inner or outer side of the ankle and foot. It's often an early sign of venous insufficiency and can be associated with more severe varicose veins.

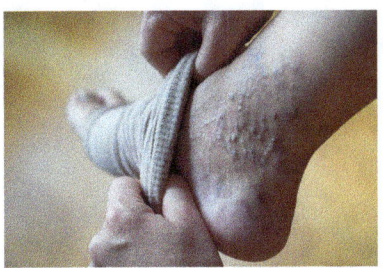

Understanding the different types of varicose veins is crucial for several reasons:

Accurate Diagnosis: Identifying the specific type of varicose vein helps healthcare providers make an accurate diagnosis and determine the most appropriate treatment plan.

Treatment Selection: Different types of varicose veins may require different treatment approaches. For example, spider veins might be treated with sclerotherapy, while larger trunk varicose veins might require more invasive procedures.

Risk Assessment: Some types of varicose veins, such as those associated with deep vein thrombosis, may pose more significant health risks and require immediate medical attention.

Patient Education: Understanding the type of varicose veins they have can help patients better comprehend their condition and make informed decisions about their treatment options.

Prognosis: The type of varicose vein can often indicate the severity of the underlying venous insufficiency and help predict the likely progression of the condition.

PART FOUR
RISK FACTORS FOR VARICOSITY

Understanding the risk factors for varicosity is crucial for both prevention and early intervention. These risk factors can increase an individual's likelihood of developing varicose veins. It's important to note that having one or more risk factors doesn't necessarily mean a person will develop varicose veins, but it does increase their chances.

AGE AND GENDER

Age

Advancing age is a significant risk factor for developing varicosity. As we age, our veins naturally lose elasticity and the valves within them may weaken.

This natural wear and tear on veins over time increases the risk of valve dysfunction, leading to blood pooling and vein dilation. The risk of developing varicose veins increases significantly after the age of 50.

However, it's important to note that varicose veins can occur at any age, including in young adults and even children in some cases.

Gender

Women are more likely to develop varicose veins than men. Studies suggest that women are two to three times more likely to develop varicosities compared to men. Several factors contribute to this increased risk in women:

a) Hormonal influences:

Female hormones, particularly estrogen and progesterone, can affect vein walls and valves. These hormones can cause vein walls to relax and dilate, potentially leading to valve dysfunction. Hormonal fluctuations during menstrual cycles, pregnancy, and menopause can further increase the risk.

b) Pregnancy:

Pregnancy significantly increases the risk of developing varicose veins. The increased blood volume during pregnancy puts additional pressure on the veins. The growing uterus can also compress pelvic veins, impeding blood flow from the legs. Hormonal changes during pregnancy contribute to vein relaxation. Varicose veins that develop during pregnancy may improve after childbirth, but often recur with subsequent pregnancies.

c) Hormonal medications:

The use of hormonal contraceptives or hormone replacement therapy can increase the risk of varicose veins in some women. While women are at higher risk, it's important to note that men can also develop varicose veins, especially if they have other risk factors.

GENETICS AND FAMILY HISTORY

Genetic predisposition:
There is a strong genetic component to the development of varicose veins. Inherited factors can affect the structural integrity of veins and the efficiency of venous valves. Specific genetic variations associated with varicose veins have been identified in recent research.

Family history:
Having a close family member (parent, sibling) with varicose veins significantly increases an individual's risk. Studies suggest that if both parents have varicose veins, the risk of developing them can be as high as 90%. If one parent has varicose veins, the risk is around 45%. The genetic influence may be related to inherited traits affecting vein wall strength, valve function, or overall vascular health.

Inherited conditions:

Certain inherited conditions that affect connective tissue, such as Ehlers-Danlos syndrome, can increase the risk of developing varicose veins. These conditions may affect the structural integrity of vein walls, making them more prone to dilation and valve dysfunction.

Ethnic considerations:

While varicose veins can affect people of all ethnicities, some studies suggest variations in prevalence among different ethnic groups. These differences may be due to a combination of genetic factors and lifestyle influences.

LIFESTYLE FACTORS

Lifestyle factors play a significant role in the development and progression of varicose veins. These factors often interact with genetic predispositions and other risk factors to increase the likelihood of developing varicosities.

Prolonged standing or sitting:

Occupations or lifestyles that require long periods of standing or sitting can increase the risk of varicose veins. Standing for extended periods increases hydrostatic pressure in the leg veins. Prolonged sitting, especially with legs crossed, can impede blood flow and increase pressure in the veins. Examples of high-risk occupations include teachers, nurses, factory workers, and office workers with sedentary jobs.

Lack of physical activity:

A sedentary lifestyle contributes to poor circulation and weakens the calf muscles. Regular exercise, especially activities that engage the calf muscles, helps promote healthy blood flow in the legs. Lack of exercise can lead to weight gain, which is another risk factor for varicose veins.

Obesity:

Being overweight or obese puts additional pressure on the veins, particularly in the legs. Excess weight can compress veins and impede blood flow. Obesity is often associated with a sedentary lifestyle, compounding the risk.

Diet:

A diet low in fiber can lead to chronic constipation, which increases abdominal pressure and can affect venous return from the legs. Inadequate intake of certain nutrients, such as vitamin C and flavonoids, may affect vein health. High-sodium diets can contribute to fluid retention, potentially increasing pressure on veins.

Smoking:

Smoking damages blood vessels and impairs circulation. It can weaken vein walls and contribute to valve dysfunction. The coughing associated with smoking can also increase intra-abdominal pressure, affecting venous return.

Tight clothing:

Wearing tight clothing, especially around the waist, groin, or legs, can restrict blood flow. This restriction can increase pressure in the veins of the legs, potentially leading to varicosities.

High heels:

Regularly wearing high heels can affect the natural functioning of the calf muscles. This can impede the efficiency of the calf muscle pump, which is crucial for helping blood return from the legs to the heart.

Sun exposure:

Excessive sun exposure, particularly to the legs, can damage small blood vessels in the skin. This damage can contribute to the development of spider veins, a type of small varicose vein.

Alcohol consumption:

Excessive alcohol intake can lead to peripheral vasodilation, potentially exacerbating existing varicose veins. Alcohol can also contribute to dehydration, which may affect overall vascular health.

MEDICAL CONDITIONS

Various medical conditions can increase the risk of developing varicose veins or exacerbate existing ones. These conditions often affect vein function, blood flow, or overall vascular health.

Chronic venous insufficiency:
This condition impairs the ability of veins to return blood efficiently to the heart. It can lead to increased venous pressure, resulting in the enlargement and twisting of veins. Chronic venous insufficiency often precedes the development of visible varicose veins.

Deep vein thrombosis (DVT):
A history of DVT can damage vein valves and impair circulation. This damage can lead to post-thrombotic syndrome, which often includes the development of varicose veins.

Phlebitis:

Inflammation of the veins, whether superficial or deep, can damage vein walls and valves. This damage can contribute to the development of varicosities.

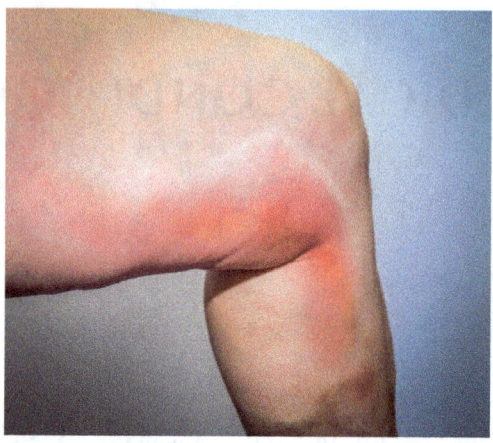

Constipation:

Chronic constipation increases intra-abdominal pressure. This increased pressure can impede venous return from the legs, potentially leading to varicose veins.

Tumors:

Pelvic or abdominal tumors can compress veins, obstructing blood flow and potentially leading to varicosities.

Arteriovenous malformations:

These abnormal connections between arteries and veins can affect blood flow and contribute to the development of varicose veins.

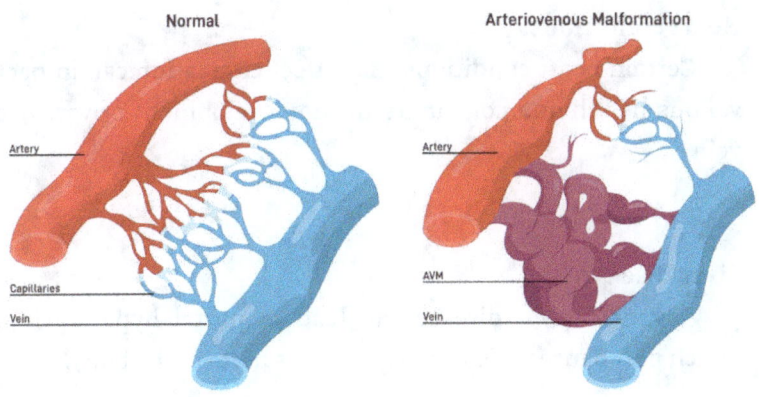

Connective tissue disorders:

Conditions like Ehlers-Danlos syndrome can affect the structural integrity of vein walls, increasing the risk of varicosities.

Hypertension:

High blood pressure can put additional stress on blood vessels, potentially contributing to vein damage and varicosity.

Heart conditions:

Certain heart conditions that affect circulation can impact venous health and contribute to the development of varicose veins.

Liver disease:

Advanced liver disease can lead to portal hypertension, which may cause varicosities in various parts of the body.

Hormonal imbalances:

Conditions affecting hormone levels, such as thyroid disorders or polycystic ovary syndrome, may influence vein health and the development of varicosities.

PART FIVE
SIGNS AND SYMPTOMS

Varicose veins can manifest with a wide range of signs and symptoms, varying in severity from person to person. Some individuals may experience only mild discomfort or cosmetic concerns, while others may suffer from more severe symptoms and complications. Understanding these signs and symptoms is crucial for early detection and proper management of varicose veins.

VISUAL INDICATORS

Visual indicators are often the first noticeable signs of varicose veins. These visible changes in the appearance of veins can range from subtle to quite prominent.

Enlarged, twisted veins:

The most characteristic visual sign of varicose veins is the appearance of enlarged, twisted, or bulging veins beneath the skin's surface. These veins typically appear rope-like or cord-like and may be raised above the skin level. They are most commonly found on the legs, particularly on the backs of the calves or along the inside of the legs. Even when veins are not significantly enlarged, they may become more visible through the skin.

This increased visibility can be due to the veins becoming more superficial or the skin becoming thinner.

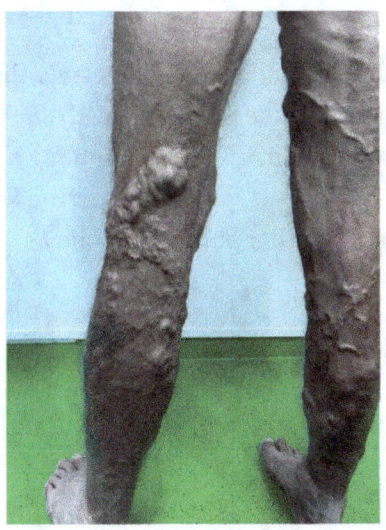

In addition to being enlarged, varicose veins may appear tortuous, meaning they have an irregular, winding shape. This distortion is often more noticeable when standing.

Color changes:
Varicose veins often appear blue, purple, or dark red. The color may be more pronounced when standing or when the affected limb is in a dependent position. In some cases, the skin over the varicose veins may take on a bluish tint.

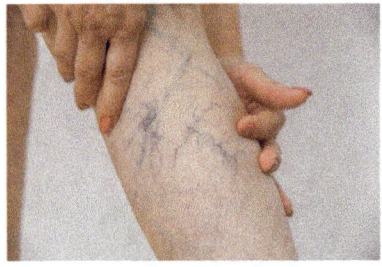

Spider veins:

These are smaller, dilated blood vessels that appear close to the skin's surface. Spider veins typically look like a network of red, purple, or blue lines, often resembling a spider's web or tree branches. They are usually found on the legs but can also appear on the face or other parts of the body.

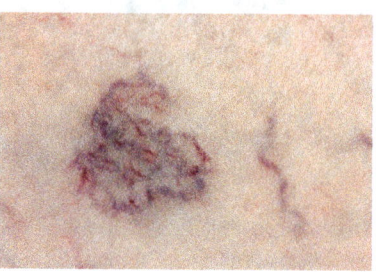

Asymmetry:

Varicose veins may cause visible asymmetry between the legs, with one leg appearing more swollen or having more prominent veins than the other.

Skin discoloration:

The skin over varicose veins may develop a brownish or reddish discoloration. This discoloration is often a sign of chronic venous insufficiency and can be an early indicator of more serious complications.

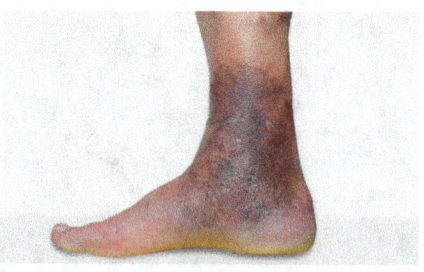

Visible ulcers:

In advanced cases, open sores or ulcers may develop, typically around the ankles or lower legs. These ulcers are usually a sign of severe venous insufficiency and require immediate medical attention.

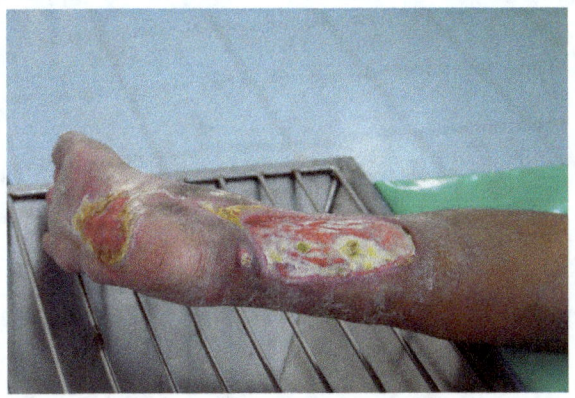

Varicose eczema:

The skin around varicose veins may become red, dry, and itchy, a condition known as varicose eczema or stasis dermatitis. This skin change is often accompanied by scaling and may lead to skin breakdown if left untreated.

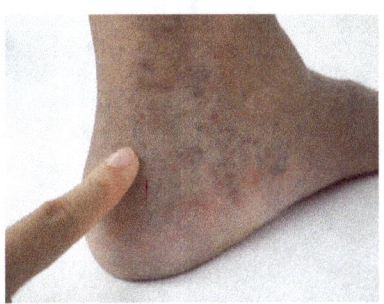

Lipodermatosclerosis:

In chronic cases, the skin and tissues around varicose veins may become hardened and contracted. This can give the lower leg a characteristic "inverted champagne bottle" appearance.

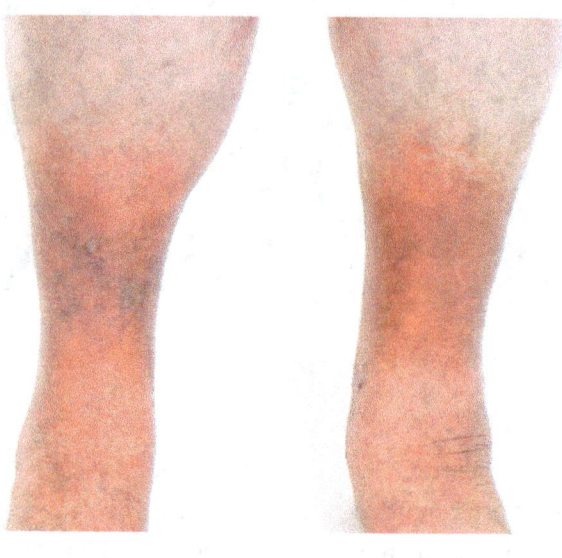

PHYSICAL DISCOMFORT AND PAIN

Varicosity is not just a cosmetic concern; it often comes with various physical symptoms that can range from mild discomfort to significant pain:

a) Aching and Heaviness: Many individuals with varicose veins experience a dull, aching sensation in their legs. This is often accompanied by a feeling of heaviness or fatigue, especially after long periods of standing or sitting.

b) Throbbing and Cramping: Varicose veins can cause a throbbing sensation in the affected areas. Some people also experience muscle cramping, particularly in the calves, which can be more pronounced at night.

c) Itching and Burning: The affected areas may feel itchy or have a burning sensation. This discomfort is often exacerbated by touch or pressure on the varicose veins.

d) Pain Worsened by Prolonged Standing or Sitting: The discomfort associated with varicose veins typically worsens after long periods of standing or sitting. This is due to increased pressure in the veins when in these positions.

e) Relief with Elevation: Many individuals find that

elevating their legs provides temporary relief from the pain and discomfort associated with varicose veins. This is because elevation helps improve blood flow and reduces pressure in the affected veins.

f) Restless Legs: Some people with varicosity experience restless leg syndrome, characterized by an uncomfortable urge to move the legs, especially at night. This can interfere with sleep and overall quality of life.

g) Tenderness: The areas around varicose veins may be tender to touch. This tenderness can range from mild to severe and may limit physical activities or affect daily routines.

SKIN CHANGES AND COMPLICATIONS

As varicosity progresses, it can lead to various skin changes and potentially serious complications:

a) Edema (Swelling): One of the most common skin changes associated with varicosity is edema or swelling. This typically occurs in the ankles and feet and may worsen throughout the day or in hot weather. The swelling is caused by fluid leaking from the dilated veins into the surrounding tissues.

b) Skin Discoloration: Chronic venous insufficiency can lead to skin discoloration in the affected areas. The skin may take on a brownish or reddish hue, a condition known as stasis dermatitis. This discoloration is due to the deposition of hemosiderin, a breakdown product of red blood cells, in the skin.

c) Dry and Itchy Skin: The skin over varicose veins often becomes dry, flaky, and itchy. This can lead to persistent scratching, which may further damage the skin and increase the risk of infection.

d) Eczema: Some individuals with varicosity develop

eczema in the affected areas. This presents as red, itchy, and inflamed patches of skin that may become scaly or crusty.

e) Lipodermatosclerosis: In advanced cases, the skin and subcutaneous tissues may become hardened and contracted, a condition known as lipodermatosclerosis. This can cause the lower leg to take on an inverted champagne bottle appearance.

f) Venous Ulcers: One of the most serious complications of varicosity is the development of venous ulcers. These are open sores that typically occur near the ankles and are characterized by their slow healing nature. Venous ulcers can be painful, prone to infection, and may significantly impact an individual's quality of life.

g) Superficial Thrombophlebitis: This condition occurs when a blood clot forms in a superficial vein, causing inflammation. It presents as a tender, warm, and reddened area along the course of a varicose vein.

h) Deep Vein Thrombosis (DVT): Although less common, varicosity can increase the risk of DVT, a serious condition where blood clots form in the deep veins of the legs. DVT requires immediate medical attention as it can lead to life-threatening complications such as pulmonary embolism.

i) Bleeding: In severe cases, varicose veins close to the skin's surface may burst, causing significant bleeding. This is more likely to occur with minor injuries or increased pressure in the veins.

j) Cellulitis: The compromised skin integrity associated with varicosity can increase the risk of cellulitis, a bacterial skin infection that can spread rapidly if left untreated.

Understanding these signs and symptoms is crucial for early identification and management of varicosity. While some individuals may experience only mild symptoms, others may face more severe complications. Regular monitoring and timely intervention can help prevent the progression of varicosity and improve overall vein health. If you notice any of these signs or symptoms, it's important to consult with a healthcare professional for proper evaluation and treatment.

PART SIX
DIAGNOSIS OF VARICOSITY

The diagnostic process for varicosity typically begins with a comprehensive medical history and thorough physical examination. This initial step is crucial in understanding the patient's symptoms, risk factors, and overall health status.

Medical History and Physical Examination

Medical History

During the medical history assessment, the healthcare provider will inquire about:

- **Symptoms:** The patient will be asked to describe their symptoms in detail, including any pain, discomfort, swelling, or visible changes in their veins. The provider will also ask about the duration and severity of these symptoms.
- **Family History:** Since varicosity can have a genetic component, the healthcare provider will ask about any family history of varicose veins or other venous disorders.
- **Risk Factors:** The patient will be questioned about potential risk factors such as age, gender, pregnancy history, occupation (especially those involving prolonged standing or sitting), obesity, and lifestyle habits.

- **Previous Treatments:** Information about any previous treatments for varicose veins or other vascular conditions will be collected.
- **Medical Conditions:** The healthcare provider will inquire about other medical conditions that might affect vein health, such as deep vein thrombosis, phlebitis, or cardiovascular diseases.

Physical Examination

The physical examination is a critical component of diagnosing varicosity. It typically involves:

- **Visual Inspection:** The healthcare provider will carefully examine the patient's legs and other potentially affected areas for visible signs of varicose veins, such as bulging or twisted veins, swelling, or skin changes.
- **Palpation:** The provider will gently feel the affected areas to assess for tenderness, warmth, or hardening of the veins.
- **Positioning Tests:** The patient may be asked to stand, sit, and change positions to observe how these changes affect the appearance of the veins and any associated symptoms.
- **Trendelenburg Test:** This test involves elevating the patient's legs and then quickly standing them up. It helps assess the competency of the venous valves.
- **Percussion Test:** The healthcare provider may tap

along the course of the veins to assess for reflux or backflow of blood.
- **Measurement:** In some cases, the circumference of the legs may be measured to quantify any swelling.

QUESTIONNAIRES FOR CHRONIC VENOUS DISEASE

Questionnaires play a crucial role in the assessment and management of chronic venous disease, including varicosity. These tools help standardize the evaluation of symptoms, quality of life impact, and disease progression. They are valuable for both initial assessment and monitoring treatment outcomes. Here are some of the most widely used and validated questionnaires for chronic venous disease:

Chronic Venous Insufficiency Questionnaire (CIVIQ)

The Chronic Venous Insufficiency Questionnaire (CIVIQ) is a validated tool designed specifically to measure the quality of life in patients suffering from chronic venous insufficiency (CVI). The CIVIQ usually consists of multiple-choice questions divided into several domains that assess different aspects of a patient's life affected by chronic venous insufficiency. These domains often include:

1. **Physical Symptoms:** Questions in this section are focused on the physical manifestations of CVI such as leg pain, swelling, cramps, and sensations of heaviness or fatigue in the legs.
2. **Psychological Well-being:** This section assesses emotional impacts, including feelings of distress or frustration due to the condition.
3. **Social Impact:** Questions here may relate to how CVI affects social interactions and daily activities, such as standing or walking for long periods, and the ability to participate in social events or work.
4. **Overall Quality of Life:** This may include broader questions about the overall impact of CVI on the patient's life satisfaction and general health perception.

Scoring the Chronic Venous Insufficiency Questionnaire (CIVIQ) generally involves a detailed process, but it's not just a simple summation of response values. The CIVIQ uses a Likert scale for its responses, and each question's score contributes to an overall score that reflects the severity of symptoms and their impact on quality of life.

Scoring Procedure:

- **Likert Scale:** Each item in the CIVQ is typically rated on a Likert scale. Commonly, these scales might range from 0 to 4 or 1 to 5, where lower scores might indicate no impact or symptom and higher scores indicate a severe impact or symptom.
- **Domain Scores:** The CIVIQ is divided into domains (e.g., physical symptoms, psychological impact,

social functioning). Each domain's score is calculated by summing the scores of the questions within that domain.
- **Weighting (if applicable):** In some versions or adaptations of the CIVIQ, certain questions or domains may be weighted differently depending on their perceived impact on quality of life. This is not always the case, but it's important to check if specific weighting rules apply to the questionnaire version being used.
- **Total Score:** The total score is typically the sum of all domain scores. This total gives an overall measure of the impact of chronic venous insufficiency on the patient's quality of life.
- **Normalization:** In some cases, scores might be normalized or adjusted based on the maximum possible score to provide a score from 0 to 100, where 100 represents the best possible quality of life and 0 represents the worst. This step involves calculating a proportion or percentage based on the total score achieved versus the total possible score.
- **Interpretation:** The final score needs to be interpreted in the context of the specific patient and the known ranges of CIVIQ scores. Higher scores typically indicate a greater impact of CVI on quality of life. Normative data or cut-off scores might be used to categorize the severity of impact.

Aberdeen Varicose Vein Questionnaire (AVVQ)

The Aberdeen Varicose Vein Questionnaire (AVVQ) is a health-related quality of life instrument specifically developed to assess the symptoms and impact of varicose veins on patients. It was developed in the 1990s by researchers at the University of Aberdeen, and it is widely used in both clinical settings and research to evaluate the burden of varicose veins from the patient's perspective.

Here is a general overview of how such a questionnaire might be scored:

- **Item Scores:** Each question in the AVVQ is typically assigned a score based on the severity or frequency of the symptom or issue being assessed. These scores are usually on a Likert scale, where higher scores indicate greater severity or impact.
- **Summing Scores:** The total score of the questionnaire is often calculated by summing the scores of all the individual items. This total score represents the overall impact of varicose veins on the patient's quality of life.
- **Weighted Scores:** In some versions of the questionnaire, different sections or specific questions might be weighted differently depending on their importance or relevance to the overall impact of the condition. This means that some aspects of the questionnaire might contribute more to the total score than others.
- **Normalization:** In certain applications, scores might be normalized or adjusted based on a scale to provide a clearer interpretation relative to a normative or baseline population. This helps in

comparing scores across different groups or conditions.
- Interpretation: The final score is interpreted to assess the severity of the condition. Higher scores typically indicate a greater impact on quality of life, more severe symptoms, or greater cosmetic concern. These scores can be used to track changes over time, especially before and after interventions.

Venous Clinical Severity Score (VCSS)

The Venous Clinical Severity Score (VCSS) is a clinical tool used to assess the severity of chronic venous disorders. It was developed as a more detailed and specific tool compared to its predecessor, the CEAP classification (Clinical, Etiologic, Anatomic, and Pathophysiologic classification), which is used to categorize venous disease.

VCSS Questionnaire Format

Pain
- 0 = None
- 1 = Mild discomfort or pain
- 2 = Moderate pain, occasional analgesics required
- 3 = Severe pain, daily analgesics required

Varicose Veins
- 0 = Absent
- 1 = Few
- 2 = Confined to calf or thigh
- 3 = Extensive (involving calf and thigh)

Venous Edema
- 0 = None
- 1 = Mild
- 2 = Moderate
- 3 = Severe

Skin Pigmentation
- 0 = None
- 1 = Mild
- 2 = Moderate
- 3 = Severe

Inflammation
0 = None
1 = Mild
2 = Moderate
3 = Severe

Induration
0 = None
1 = Mild
2 = Moderate
3 = Severe

Number of Active Ulcers
0 = None
1 = 1 ulcer
2 = 2 ulcers
3 = 3 or more ulcers

Duration of Active Ulcer (longest active ulcer)
0 = None
1 = <3 months
2 = 3 to 12 months
3 = >12 months

Size of Active Ulcer (largest ulcer)
0 = None
1 = <2 cm in diameter
2 = 2 to 6 cm in diameter
3 = >6 cm in diameter

Compression Therapy (use and compliance)
0 = Not indicated or full compliance
1 = Inconsistent use

2 = Refusal or inability to wear compression

Each parameter is scored from 0 to 3 based on the severity or status of the condition. The sum of these scores provides a composite score that reflects the overall severity of the chronic venous disease. This score can help guide treatment decisions and monitor changes in the condition over time.

Steps to Score the VCSS

Assess Each Category:
Each of the 10 categories (Pain, Varicose Veins, Venous Edema, Skin Pigmentation, Inflammation, Induration, Number of Active Ulcers, Duration of Active Ulcer, Size of Active Ulcer, and Compression Therapy) is assessed and given a score from 0 to 3. The scoring for each category is based on the severity or the presence of specific characteristics as defined in the questionnaire.

Sum the Scores:
Add up the individual scores from each of the 10 categories. The total can range from 0 (no signs of severity in any category) to 30 (maximum severity in all categories).

Interpretation

1. A higher total score indicates a more severe condition.
2. The score helps in tracking the progression of the disease or the response to treatment.

3. Regular assessments can be useful in adjusting treatment plans based on changes in the VCSS score.

Venous Insufficiency Epidemiological and Economic Study – Quality of Life/Symptoms (VEINES-QOL/Sym)

The Venous Insufficiency Epidemiological and Economic Study – Quality of Life/Symptoms (VEINES-QOL/Sym) is a validated questionnaire specifically designed to assess the quality of life and symptoms related to chronic venous disorders of the leg.

Structure of the VEINES-QOL/Sym Questionnaire

The VEINES-QOL/Sym typically includes the following types of items:

Symptom Assessment:
Frequency and intensity of leg pain, cramps, and heaviness.
Occurrence of swelling and its impact on daily activities.
Presence of skin changes or ulcers.

Quality of Life Assessment:
Impact of symptoms on daily activities (e.g., walking, standing).
Emotional impact, including feelings of frustration or embarrassment.
Social and occupational effects, such as limitations at work or in social interactions.

Overall Health Perception:
General health status.
Comparison of health to others.

Scoring Process

Each response option for the questionnaire items is assigned a numerical value. Typically, these values are scaled to reflect the severity or frequency of symptoms or the impact on quality of life, with higher scores often representing a greater impact or more frequent symptoms. The scores for individual questions are summed to produce a total score or scores for different subscales. In some cases, scores might be normalized or standardized based on sample or population norms. This can help in comparing scores across different populations or age groups. The final scores are interpreted based on established thresholds or norms that indicate the severity of symptoms or the impact on quality of life. Higher scores on symptom scales typically indicate worse symptoms, while higher scores on quality of life scales usually reflect poorer quality of life.

Special Considerations

- **Thresholds for Clinical Significance:** There might be specific thresholds established that indicate when a score is considered clinically significant, which can guide interventions.
- **Comparative Scores:** Scores might also be used to compare pre- and post-treatment conditions in clinical trials or to evaluate the effectiveness of a particular treatment or intervention over time.

When selecting a questionnaire for use in clinical practice or research, it's important to consider factors such as the specific focus of the questionnaire, its validation in relevant populations, and its sensitivity to change. Often, a combination of clinician-assessed measures (like VCSS) and patient-reported outcomes (like CIVIQ or AVVQ) provides the most comprehensive assessment of a patient's condition.

By incorporating these questionnaires into the diagnostic and management process, healthcare providers can gain a more holistic understanding of how chronic venous disease affects their patients, leading to more personalized and effective care

DIAGNOSTIC TESTS AND IMAGING

While the medical history, physical examination and using various questionnaires provide valuable information, additional diagnostic tests and imaging studies are often necessary to confirm the diagnosis, assess the extent of the condition, and plan appropriate treatment.

Doppler Ultrasound

Doppler ultrasound is the gold standard for diagnosing varicosity and assessing venous function. This non-invasive imaging technique uses sound waves to visualize blood flow within the veins and evaluate the structure and function of venous valves.

Procedure: A handheld device called a transducer is moved over the skin, emitting sound waves that bounce off blood cells and create images on a monitor.

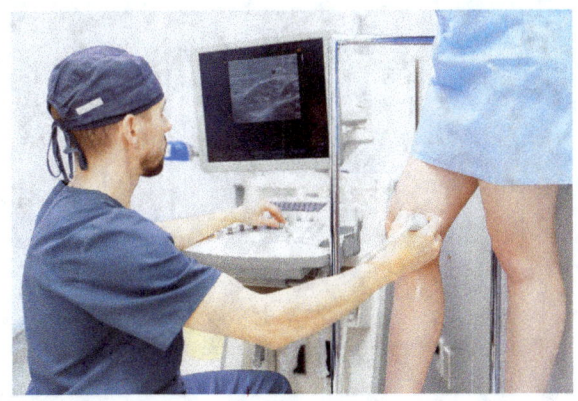

Doppler ultrasound can identify the location and extent of varicose veins, assess blood flow direction and velocity, evaluate the function of venous valves, and detect blood clots or other vascular abnormalities.

Venography

While less commonly used due to the effectiveness of ultrasound, venography may be employed in certain cases.

Procedure: A contrast dye is injected into the veins, and X-rays are taken to visualize the venous system. Venography provides detailed images of the deep venous system and can identify obstructions or abnormalities not visible through ultrasound.

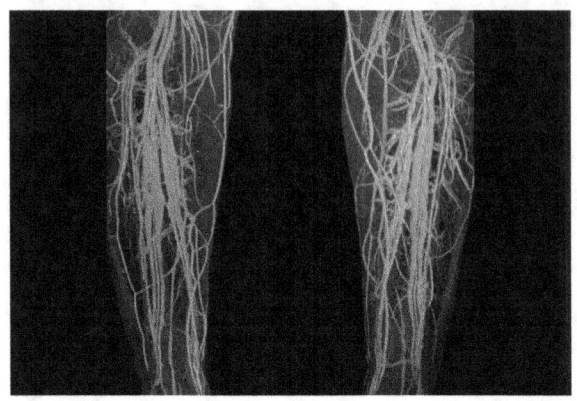

Limitations: It's an invasive procedure and carries a small risk of complications related to the contrast dye.

CT Venography

Computed Tomography (CT) venography combines CT scanning with intravenous contrast to provide detailed images of the venous system.

Benefits: Offers high-resolution, three-dimensional images of the veins, which can be particularly useful in complex cases or when planning surgical interventions.

MR Venography

Magnetic Resonance (MR) venography uses magnetic fields and radio waves to create detailed images of the venous system.

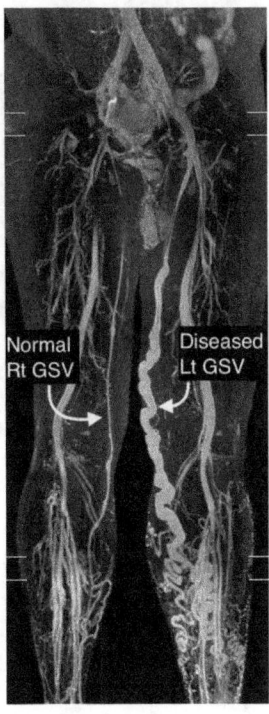

Benefits: Provides high-quality images without radiation exposure and can be particularly useful for assessing pelvic veins or in patients who cannot receive iodine-based contrast.

Plethysmography

This test measures changes in blood volume in the legs and can help assess venous function.

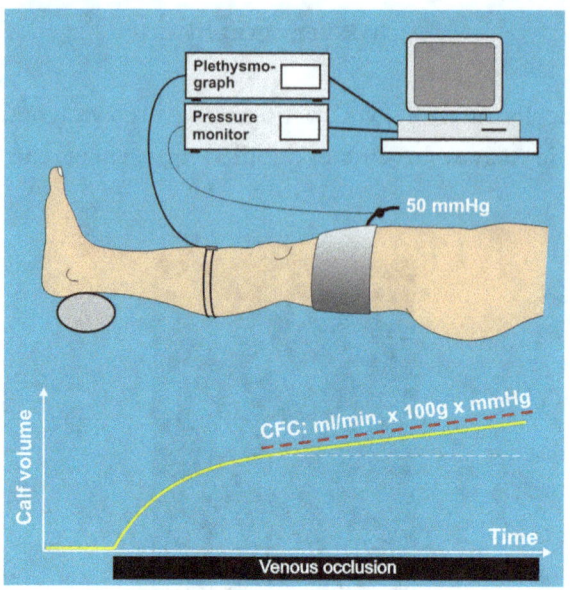

Types:

- Air Plethysmography: Measures changes in leg volume using air-filled cuffs
- Photoplethysmography: Uses infrared light to measure blood flow in the skin

The choice of diagnostic tests depends on various factors, including the severity of symptoms, the suspected extent of the condition, and the availability of specific technologies. Often, a combination of these diagnostic methods is used to obtain a comprehensive understanding of the patient's venous health.

The results of these diagnostic tests are interpreted by specialists who consider:

- The location and extent of varicose veins
- The presence of venous reflux (backward flow of blood)
- The competency of venous valves
- Any signs of deep vein thrombosis or other vascular abnormalities
- The overall function of the venous system

Based on these findings, healthcare providers can develop an appropriate treatment plan tailored to the individual patient's needs. The diagnosis of varicosity is not just about identifying the presence of varicose veins but also understanding their underlying causes, extent, and potential complications. This comprehensive approach ensures that patients receive the most effective and appropriate treatment for their specific condition.

PART SEVEN
CONSERVATIVE MANAGEMENT STRATEGIES

Conservative management strategies are often the first line of treatment for varicosity. These approaches aim to alleviate symptoms, prevent progression of the condition, and improve overall vein health without resorting to invasive procedures. The three main pillars of conservative management are lifestyle modifications, compression therapy, and exercise combined with leg elevation.

LIFESTYLE MODIFICATIONS

Lifestyle modifications play a crucial role in managing varicosity and can significantly improve symptoms and slow the progression of the condition. These changes often focus on addressing risk factors and improving overall circulatory health.

Weight Management

Maintaining a healthy weight is essential for managing varicosity. Excess weight puts additional pressure on the veins, particularly in the legs, which can exacerbate varicose veins.

Balanced Diet: Adopting a balanced, nutrient-rich diet can help in weight management. Focus on:

- Fiber-rich foods to promote healthy digestion and

prevent constipation, which can worsen varicose veins
- Foods high in flavonoids (like berries, citrus fruits, and leafy greens) to support vein health
- Adequate hydration to maintain blood volume and prevent blood thickening

Regular Exercise: Incorporate regular physical activity to maintain a healthy weight. Low-impact exercises like walking, swimming, or cycling can be particularly beneficial for individuals with varicosity.

Avoiding Prolonged Standing or Sitting

Prolonged periods of standing or sitting can increase pressure in the veins and worsen varicosity symptoms.

Frequent Movement: If your job requires long periods of standing or sitting, try to take frequent breaks to move around or change position.

Elevate Feet: When sitting for extended periods, elevate your feet to promote blood flow back to the heart.

Standing Desk: Consider using a standing desk that allows you to alternate between sitting and standing throughout the day.

Clothing Choices

Certain clothing choices can impact vein health and varicosity symptoms.

Avoid Tight Clothing: Tight clothes, especially around the waist, groin, or legs, can restrict blood flow and exacerbate varicosity.

Comfortable Footwear: Choose comfortable, low-heeled shoes that support the calf muscles and promote good circulation.

Smoking Cessation

Smoking can damage blood vessels and impair circulation, potentially worsening varicosity.

Seek Support: If you smoke, consider seeking support to quit. This can significantly improve your overall vascular health.

Managing Other Health Conditions

Certain health conditions can impact vein health and should be properly managed.

Blood Pressure Control: High blood pressure can put additional stress on veins. Work with your healthcare provider to keep your blood pressure within a healthy range.

Hormone Management: For women, hormonal changes (such as during pregnancy or menopause) can affect vein health. Discuss hormone management strategies with your healthcare provider if necessary.

COMPRESSION THERAPY

Compression stockings are specially designed garments that apply graduated pressure to the legs, with the greatest pressure at the ankles and decreasing pressure moving up the leg.

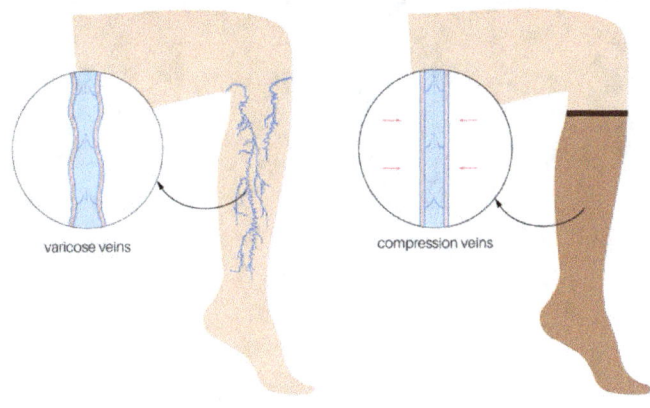

Types of Compression Stockings:

- Knee-high stockings: Most common, covering from the foot to just below the knee
- Thigh-high stockings: Extend from the foot to the upper thigh
- Pantyhose: Cover the entire lower body from the waist down

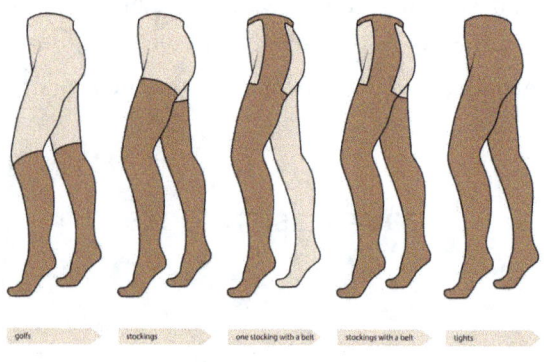

Compression Levels

Class 1: Light Compression

- **Pressure Range:** 15-20 mmHg
- **Purpose:** Ideal for mild varicose veins, slight swelling, and for relief from tired, aching legs. This class is also commonly used for travel and during pregnancy to prevent varicose veins.

Class 2: Medium Compression

- **Pressure Range:** 20-30 mmHg
- **Purpose:** Used for moderate varicose veins, moderate edema, and after healing of minor ulcers. It is also prescribed for post-surgical and post-sclerotherapy treatment to help prevent the reappearance of varicose and spider veins.

Class 3: High Compression

- **Pressure Range:** 30-40 mmHg
- **Purpose:** Suitable for severe varicose veins, severe edema, chronic venous insufficiency, and after deep vein thrombosis. This class is often recommended for more severe venous disorders.

Class 4: Extra High Compression

Pressure Range: 40-50 mmHg or more

Purpose: This class is intended for severe cases, including lymphedema and other severe swelling. It helps manage active ulcers and manifestations of post-thrombotic syndrome.

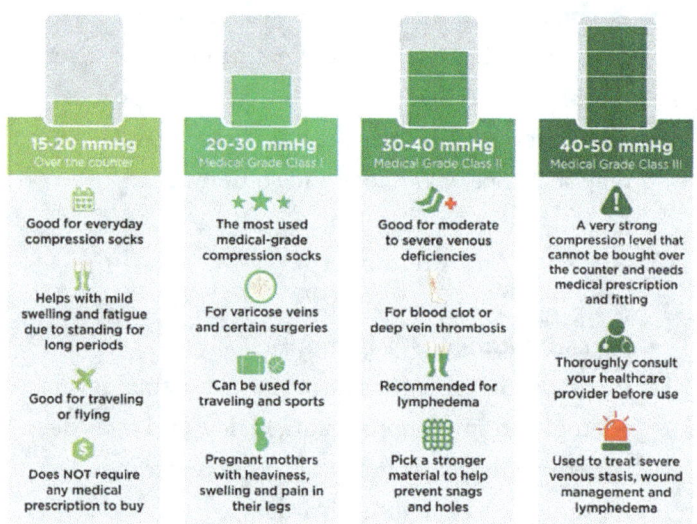

Compression Wraps

For individuals who have difficulty putting on compression stockings, compression wraps can be an alternative.

Short-stretch bandages: These provide high working pressure during muscle activity and low resting pressure.

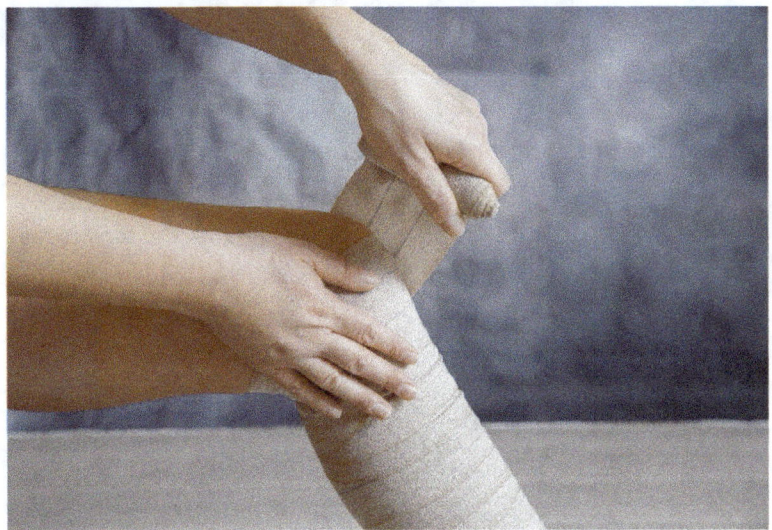

Velcro wraps: Adjustable wraps that allow for easy application and removal.

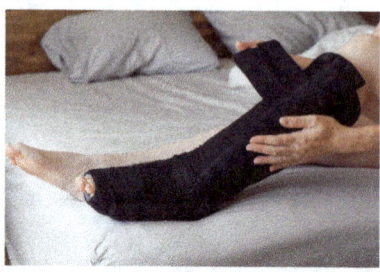

Intermittent Pneumatic Compression Devices

These devices use inflatable garments to apply intermittent pressure to the legs, mimicking the natural muscle pump action. Particularly useful for individuals with limited mobility or severe chronic venous insufficiency.

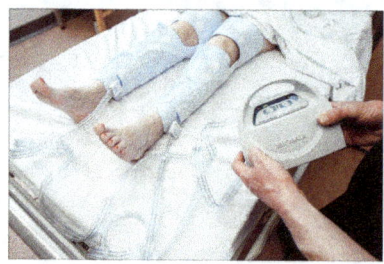

Choosing the Right Class

When selecting compression stockings, it's important to consult with a healthcare provider to ensure the appropriate class and fit. Incorrect usage can lead to further complications, so a professional assessment is crucial for effective treatment and comfort. Additionally, factors such as the length of the stocking (knee-high, thigh-high, or pantyhose) and the type (open-toe or closed-toe) are also important considerations based on the specific medical needs and lifestyle of the individual.

PHARMACOLOGICAL MANAGEMENT

While lifestyle modifications, compression therapy, and exercise form the cornerstone of conservative management for varicosity, pharmacological interventions can play a significant role in symptom relief and disease management. Various medications are available, ranging from over-the-counter options to prescription drugs, each targeting different aspects of venous insufficiency.

Venoactive Drugs (Phlebotropic Drugs)

Venoactive drugs, also known as phlebotropic drugs, are a class of medications that act on the venous system to improve venous tone, reduce inflammation, and enhance microcirculation. These drugs are widely used in Europe and are gaining acceptance in other parts of the world.

FLAVONOIDS:

Micronized Purified Flavonoid Fraction (MPFF): Contains 90% diosmin and 10% hesperidin

Mechanism: Improves venous tone, reduces inflammation, and enhances lymphatic drainage
    Dosage: Typically 500 mg twice daily
    Benefits: Reduces edema, pain, and heaviness associated with chronic venous insufficiency

RUTIN AND RUTOSIDES:

Mechanism: Improves venous tone and reduces capillary permeability
    Dosage: Varies by preparation, typically 1000-3000 mg daily
    Benefits: Reduces edema and alleviates symptoms of venous insufficiency

HORSE CHESTNUT SEED EXTRACT:

Mechanism: Active ingredient (Aescin) improves venous tone and reduces capillary permeability
    Dosage: Typically 300 mg twice daily (containing 50 mg aescin per dose)
    Benefits: Reduces leg volume and circumference, alleviates pain and itching

PYCNOGENOL (FRENCH MARITIME PINE BARK EXTRACT):

Mechanism: Potent antioxidant, improves endothelial function
Dosage: Typically 50-100 mg daily
Benefits: Reduces edema, improves skin trophic changes

CALCIUM DOBESILATE:

Mechanism: Reduces capillary permeability, improves lymphatic drainage
Dosage: Typically 500 mg twice daily
Benefits: Reduces edema, cramps, and pain associated with chronic venous insufficiency

PENTOXIFYLLINE:

While primarily used for peripheral artery disease, pentoxifylline has shown benefits in venous disease, particularly in the healing of venous ulcers.

Mechanism: Improves blood flow by increasing red blood cell flexibility and reducing blood viscosity
Dosage: Typically 400 mg three times daily
Benefits: Accelerates healing of venous ulcers when used in conjunction with compression therapy

TOPICAL AGENTS:

Various topical preparations are available for symptomatic relief and to address skin changes associated with chronic venous insufficiency.

HEPARINOID CREAMS:

Mechanism: Anti-inflammatory and antithrombotic effects
  Usage: Applied to affected areas 2-3 times daily
  Benefits: Reduces inflammation, improves microcirculation

TOPICAL CORTICOSTEROIDS:

Mechanism: Potent anti-inflammatory effect
  Usage: Short-term application for acute inflammation or severe itching
  Caution: Long-term use can lead to skin atrophy and other adverse effects

ZINC OXIDE PREPARATIONS:

Mechanism: Provides a protective barrier and promotes wound healing
  Usage: Applied to areas of skin damage or venous ulcers
  Benefits: Protects skin, promotes healing of minor wounds and irritations

ANTICOAGULANTS:

While not directly treating varicosity, anticoagulants play a crucial role in managing and preventing complications associated with chronic venous insufficiency, particularly deep vein thrombosis (DVT).

Low Molecular Weight Heparin (LMWH):
Mechanism: Inhibits blood clotting factors

Usage: Subcutaneous injection, typically for short-term prophylaxis or treatment of DVT

Benefits: Prevents formation of new blood clots and progression of existing ones

Direct Oral Anticoagulants (DOACs):
Examples: Rivaroxaban, Apixaban, Edoxaban

Mechanism: Directly inhibit specific clotting factors

Usage: Oral administration, for long-term management of DVT risk

Benefits: Convenient oral dosing, no need for regular blood monitoring

Diuretics:
While not a primary treatment for varicosity, diuretics may be prescribed in cases where edema is a significant problem and not adequately controlled by other measures.

Mechanism: Increases urine output, reducing fluid retention

Usage: Oral administration, dosage varies by specific drug

Caution: Should be used judiciously as they can lead to electrolyte imbalances and dehydration

Antibiotics:

In cases where venous ulcers become infected, systemic or topical antibiotics may be necessary.

Usage: Determined by the type and severity of infection

Importance: Proper wound care and addressing underlying venous insufficiency are crucial alongside antibiotic treatment

PAIN MANAGEMENT:

For patients experiencing significant pain associated with varicosity or venous ulcers, pain management medications may be prescribed.

Non-Steroidal Anti-Inflammatory Drugs (NSAIDs):

Mechanism: Reduces inflammation and pain

Usage: Oral or topical application

Caution: Long-term use should be monitored due to potential gastrointestinal and cardiovascular side effects

Acetaminophen (Paracetamol):

Mechanism: Pain relief without anti-inflammatory effects

Usage: Oral administration

Benefits: Generally well-tolerated for long-term use when taken as directed

Important Considerations for Pharmacological Management

Individualized Approach: The choice of medication should be tailored to the individual patient, considering the severity of their condition, comorbidities, and potential drug interactions.

Combination Therapy: Often, a combination of different medications and non-pharmacological interventions yields the best results.

Monitoring: Regular follow-ups are essential to assess the effectiveness of the medication and monitor for any side effects.

Patient Education: Patients should be educated about the proper use of medications, potential side effects, and the importance of adherence to the treatment plan.

Evidence-Based Practice: While many of these medications have shown benefits in clinical studies, the strength of evidence varies. Healthcare providers should stay updated on the latest research and guidelines.

Complementary Nature: Pharmacological management should be seen as complementary to other conservative measures like compression therapy and lifestyle modifications, not as a replacement for them.

Long-Term Management: Chronic venous insufficiency is often a long-term condition, and the treatment plan may need to be adjusted over time based on the patient's response and disease progression.

PART EIGHT
MINIMALLY INVASIVE TREATMENTS

Minimally invasive treatments for varicosity offer effective solutions with less recovery time and reduced risk compared to traditional surgery. These treatments, which include sclerotherapy, thermablation (such as endovenous laser treatment and radiofrequency ablation), and non-thermal ablation, are designed to close off problematic veins, thus alleviating symptoms and improving cosmetic appearance.

SCLEROTHERAPY

Sclerotherapy is one of the most common minimally invasive procedures for treating varicose and spider veins. This treatment involves injecting a sclerosant solution directly into the affected vein. The sclerosant irritates the lining of the vein, causing it to collapse and stick together. Over time, the treated vein scars and is reabsorbed by the body, and the blood is rerouted through healthier veins.

Liquid Sclerotherapy

- Traditional method using liquid sclerosing agents
- Best suited for small spider veins and reticular veins
- Common solutions: sodium tetradecyl sulfate, polidocanol

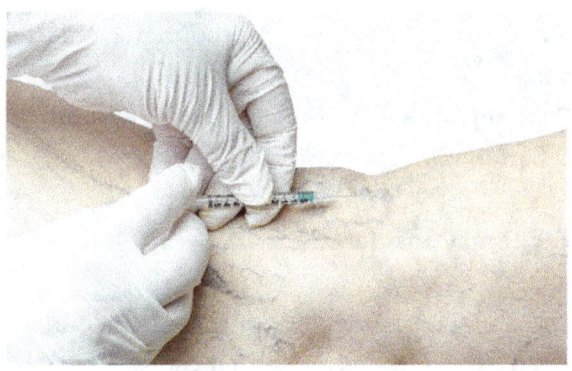

Foam Sclerotherapy

- Involves mixing the sclerosing solution with air or CO_2 to create foam
- More effective for larger veins as foam displaces blood and increases contact with vein walls
- Better visualization under ultrasound guidance

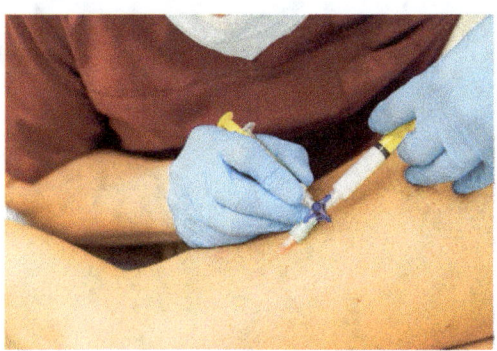

Recovery and Results

- Minimal downtime
- Compression stockings required for 1-2 weeks
- Multiple sessions may be needed

- Success rates: 60-80% for appropriately selected veins
- Possible side effects: bruising, pigmentation, inflammation

Efficacy and Considerations

- Sclerotherapy is effective for small to medium-sized varicose veins and spider veins.
- Multiple sessions may be required depending on the extent and size of the veins treated.
- Common side effects include bruising, redness, and swelling at the injection site.

THERMABLATION

Thermablation includes two primary techniques: Endovenous Laser Treatment (EVLT) and Radiofrequency Ablation (RFA). Both methods use heat to cause the affected veins to collapse.

Endovenous Laser Treatment (EVLT)

Description

EVLT uses laser energy to heat and close off varicose veins. A laser fiber is inserted into the vein through a small incision under ultrasound guidance.

Procedure

- Local anesthesia is used to numb the treatment area.

- A thin laser fiber is threaded into the vein, and laser energy is emitted to heat the vein, causing it to collapse and seal shut.

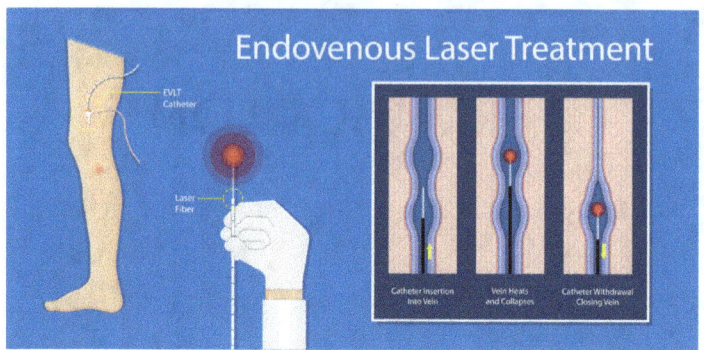

Recovery and Care

- The procedure is outpatient, with minimal downtime.
- Walking is encouraged soon after the procedure to promote circulation.
- Compression stockings are recommended for 1-2 weeks post-treatment.

Efficacy and Considerations

- EVLT is highly effective for larger varicose veins.
- It offers a 98% success rate in eliminating treated veins.
- Side effects may include temporary bruising, swelling, and discomfort.

Radiofrequency Ablation (RFA)

RFA is similar to EVLT but uses radiofrequency energy to heat the vein.

Procedure

- Local anesthesia is administered.
- A catheter is inserted into the vein, and radiofrequency energy is applied to heat and close the vein.

Recovery and Care

- Patients can usually return to normal activities the following day.
- Compression stockings are worn to support the healing process.

Efficacy and Considerations

- RFA is particularly effective for treating the great saphenous vein in the leg.
- It is associated with less pain and bruising compared to laser treatment.

NON-THERMAL ABLATION

Non-thermal ablation techniques, such as ultrasound-guided foam sclerotherapy (UGFS) and mechanochemical ablation (MOCA), use chemical or mechanical means rather than heat to close the veins.

Non-thermal ablation techniques, such as ultrasound-guided foam sclerotherapy (UGFS) and mechanochemical ablation (MOCA), use chemical or mechanical means rather than heat to close the veins.

Description and Procedure

UGFS involves injecting a foam sclerosant under ultrasound guidance, which displaces the blood and directly contacts the vein wall, causing it to collapse.

MOCA combines mechanical agitation of the vein with a sclerosant to achieve vein closure without thermal energy.

Recovery and Care

- Both procedures allow for immediate walking and quick return to daily activities.
- Compression stockings are often recommended.

Efficacy and Considerations

These methods are suitable for patients who are not good candidates for thermal ablation. They avoid the need for tumescent anesthesia, reducing discomfort and recovery time.

Each of these treatments has its specific applications, advantages, and considerations. The choice of treatment depends on the size, location, and severity of the varicose veins, as well as patient preference and medical history. Consultation with a vascular specialist or dermatologist experienced in these procedures is essential to determine the most appropriate treatment plan.

PART NINE
SURGICAL INTERVENTIONS

When conservative treatments prove insufficient or in cases of severe varicosity, surgical interventions may become necessary. These procedures offer more definitive solutions for patients experiencing significant symptoms or complications from varicose veins. Surgical approaches have evolved significantly over the years, providing various options that range from traditional vein stripping to more modern, minimally invasive techniques. These procedures offer distinct advantages and are suitable for different clinical scenarios, allowing healthcare providers to tailor the treatment approach to individual patient needs. Understanding these surgical options is crucial for both healthcare providers and patients in making informed decisions about treatment pathways.

While surgical interventions generally provide more permanent solutions compared to conservative treatments, they require careful consideration of factors such as recovery time, potential complications, and long-term outcomes. The choice of surgical approach depends on various factors, including the severity of varicosity, the location and size of affected veins, overall health status, and patient preferences.

VEIN STRIPPING

Vein stripping is an established surgical technique conducted under general anesthesia, specifically aimed at addressing severe varicose veins. This procedure is generally considered when:

- Conservative treatments have proven ineffective,
- Substantial varicose veins exist,
- Alternative therapeutic methods have failed, and
- Significant symptoms are impacting the patient's quality of life.

PROCEDURE OVERVIEW

1. Small incisions are made at both the top and bottom of the targeted vein.
2. A slim, flexible instrument known as a stripper is threaded through the vein.
3. The vein is then secured to the stripper.

4. The vein is extracted by pulling it out through one of the incisions.

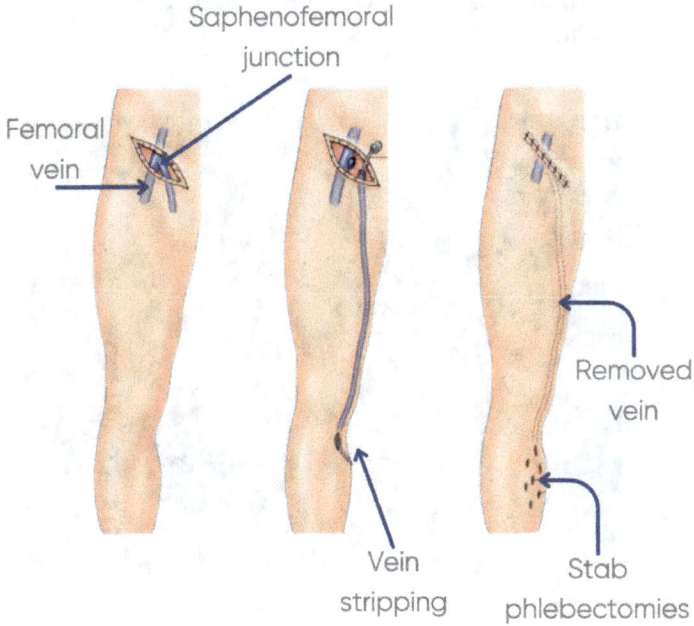

ADVANTAGES

- Immediate elimination of problematic veins,
- Durable outcomes,
- Effective in treating severe cases,
- Capability to treat multiple veins in a single session.

RECOVERY CONSIDERATIONS

- General anesthesia is required,
- A hospital stay may be necessary,

- A recovery period ranging from two to four weeks,
- Compression stockings are required during the recovery phase,
- Regular walking is recommended to facilitate healing.

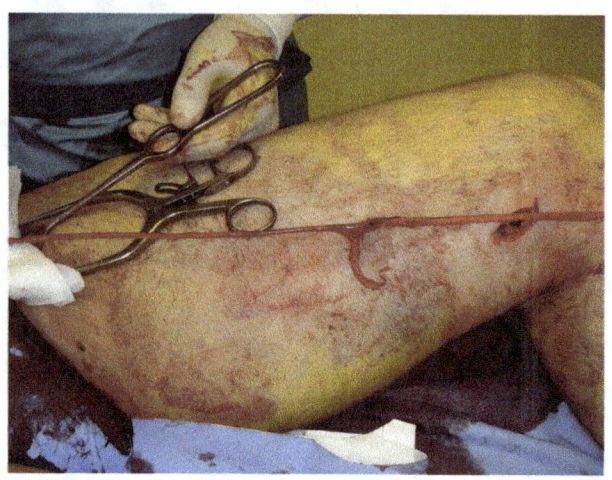

AMBULATORY PHLEBECTOMY

Ambulatory phlebectomy is a minimally invasive surgical procedure carried out under local anesthesia, designed to efficiently address specific venous conditions. It is particularly effective for:

- Removing superficial varicose veins,
- Treating clusters of varicose veins,
- Managing veins that are too large for sclerotherapy but too small for vein stripping.

PROCEDURE DETAILS

- Tiny incisions (1-2mm) are made along the targeted veins. Specialized hooks are employed to grasp and extract segments of the vein.
- Veins are removed in small sections through these micro-incisions. Multiple veins can be addressed in a single session.

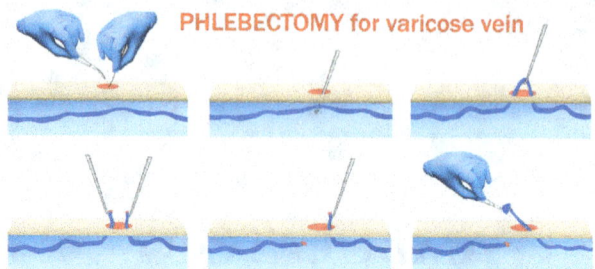

BENEFITS

- Minimal scarring due to the small size of incisions,
- Utilizes only local anesthesia,
- Outpatient procedure allowing patients to return home the same day,
- Quick recovery time facilitating a swift return to daily activities,
- Immediate visible results,
- High success rate in removing targeted veins.

RECOVERY PROCESS

- Patients are encouraged to walk immediately following the procedure to promote circulation.
- Compression stockings are required for 1-2 weeks to support recovery.
- Most daily activities can typically be resumed within 24-48 hours.
- The procedure causes minimal pain and discomfort.
- Small incisions typically heal quickly and do not require sutures.

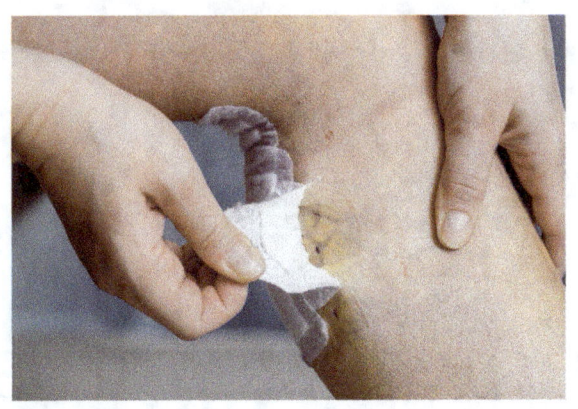

PART TEN
SPECIAL CONSIDERATIONS

VARICOSITY DURING PREGNANCY

Physiological Changes and Impact on Veins

Pregnancy induces significant physiological changes that increase the risk of developing varicosity. These include:

- **Hormonal Changes:** Increased levels of progesterone during pregnancy cause the walls of blood vessels to relax, which can lead to valve dysfunction and vein dilation.
- **Increased Blood Volume:** To support fetal development, blood volume increases by approximately 40-50%, placing additional pressure on the veins.
- **Uterine Pressure:** As the uterus grows, it can exert pressure on the inferior vena cava (a major vein returning blood from the lower body to the heart), impeding blood flow and increasing venous pressure in the legs.

Symptoms and Risks

Pregnant women might notice more pronounced vein patterns, especially in the legs and vulvar area. Symptoms can include leg heaviness, swelling, and pain. The primary risks associated with varicosity in pregnancy include thrombosis (particularly deep vein thrombosis), phlebitis, and increased risk of venous insufficiency post-pregnancy.

Management Strategies

- **Compression Therapy:** Medical-grade compression stockings can alleviate symptoms by enhancing venous return and reducing edema.
- **Regular Exercise:** Activities such as walking and prenatal yoga can improve circulation and vein health.
- **Proper Nutrition:** A balanced diet rich in vitamins C and E can support vascular health and skin integrity.
- **Elevated Leg Rest:** Elevating the legs above heart level when possible can help reduce venous pressure and swelling.
- **Regular Check-ups:** Monitoring by healthcare providers can help manage symptoms and prevent complications.

Varicosity in Athletes

Causes and Concerns

Athletes, especially those involved in high-impact sports like running or weightlifting, may experience exacerbated symptoms of varicosity due to repetitive stress and increased abdominal pressure which affect blood flow.

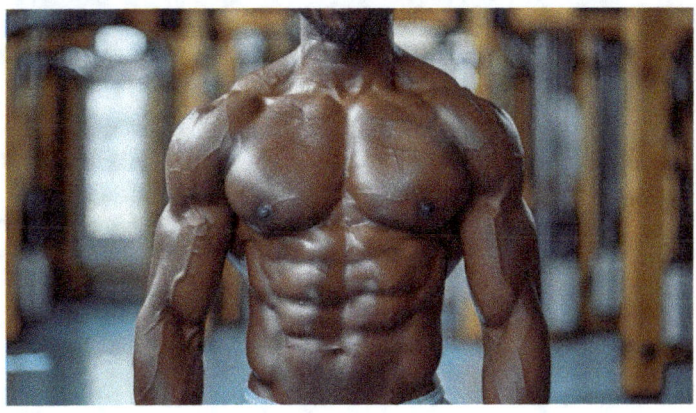

Symptoms and Complications

Symptoms in athletes often include aching, fatigue, and

swelling in the legs after long periods of exercise or standing. The main concerns for athletes with varicosity are impaired performance, increased risk of superficial vein thrombosis, and progression to chronic venous insufficiency.

Management and Prevention

- **Compression Garments:** Wearing compression socks or sleeves during and after exercise can improve blood flow and reduce symptoms.
- **Cross-Training:** Incorporating low-impact exercises such as swimming or cycling can help manage and prevent exacerbation of symptoms without sacrificing cardiovascular fitness.
- **Adequate Hydration and Nutrition:** Proper hydration and a diet rich in flavonoids and antioxidants can support vein health.
- **Proper Recovery:** Including rest days and recovery techniques such as elevation of the legs, massage, and cool-down stretches can help manage symptoms.
- **Medical Assessment:** Regular evaluations by a sports physician or a vascular specialist can help manage varicosity and prevent complications.

VARICOSITY IN HANDS AND ARMS

While varicosity is most commonly associated with the legs, visible veins can also appear on the hands and arms. This condition, although less common, can cause cosmetic concerns and, in some cases, discomfort. Understanding the causes, symptoms, and potential treatment options is essential for those experiencing this condition.

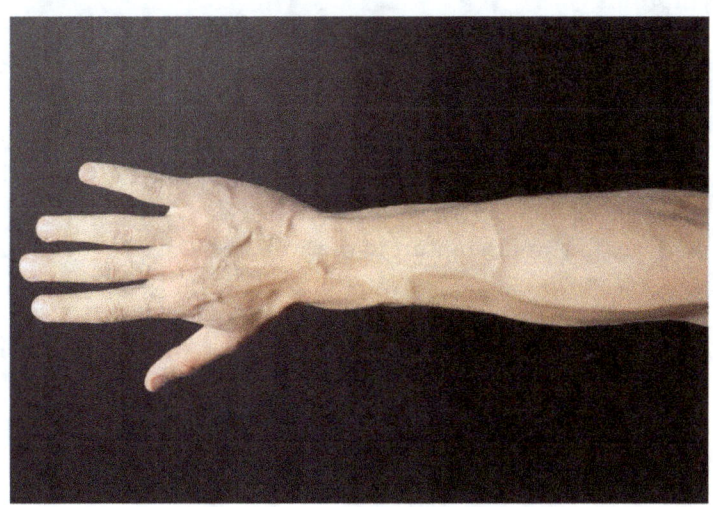

Causes and Risk Factors

Varicosity in the hands and arms can occur due to several reasons:

1 Aging: As we age, skin becomes thinner and less elastic, making veins more visible. The loss of fat and tissue structure also contributes to more prominent veins.

2 Physical Strain: Repetitive use of the arms and hands in activities like weightlifting, jobs that require manual labor, or sports that involve significant arm use can increase venous pressure and lead to varicosity.

3 Genetic Factors: Heredity plays a role in the development of varicose veins, including those on the arms and hands.

4 Hormonal Changes: Similar to leg varicosity, hormonal fluctuations can affect vein elasticity and valve functionality, contributing to varicosity.

5 Temperature Fluctuations: Exposure to extreme temperatures can cause veins to expand and contract, which may make them more visible and prone to damage.

Symptoms

The primary symptom of varicosity in the hands and arms is the visible appearance of blue or purple veins that may look twisted or bulging. While these are often asymptomatic, some individuals may experience:

- Aching or discomfort in the arms or hands
- Feeling of heaviness or fatigue in the limbs after prolonged use
- Swelling, particularly in the hands

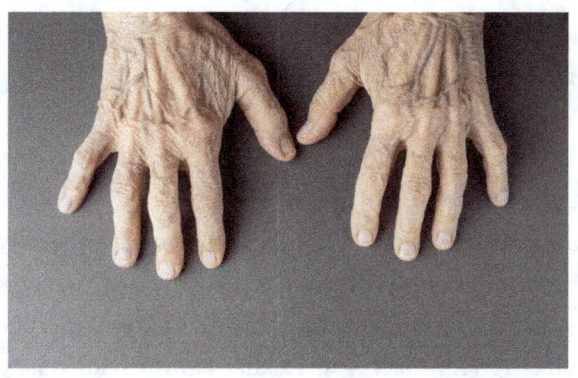

Management and Treatment

For many individuals, varicosity in the hands and arms is a cosmetic issue rather than a medical concern. However, there are several strategies to manage symptoms and improve appearance:

1 Compression Garments: Compression gloves or sleeves can help improve circulation and reduce the visibility of veins. These are particularly useful for those involved in repetitive manual activities.

2 Exercise: Regular cardiovascular and strength-training exercises can enhance circulation and vein health. Focus on exercises that improve arm strength and blood flow.

3 Elevation: Elevating the arms can help reduce venous pressure and swelling, thus diminishing the appearance of veins.

4 Skincare: Moisturizing the skin can improve its appearance and elasticity, making veins less noticeable. Use of sun protection also helps prevent skin damage and thinning.

5 Diet and Hydration: A diet rich in bioflavonoids (found in citrus fruits, berries, and green tea) can strengthen veins. Hydration is crucial as it improves blood flow and vein health.

6 Sclerotherapy: For persistent or bothersome veins, sclerotherapy, where a solution is injected into the vein causing it to collapse and fade, can be an option. This treatment is also used for larger veins.

When to Seek Medical Advice

While varicosity in the hands and arms is generally harmless, it is important to consult with a healthcare provider if there is pain, significant discomfort, or concern about the condition's appearance. A specialist can provide assessments and recommend treatments based on individual needs and the severity of the condition.

PART ELEVEN
COMPLICATIONS OF UNTREATED VARICOSITY

Varicosity, commonly known as varicose veins, if left untreated, can lead to several serious health complications. This section delves into the progression of untreated varicosity into more severe conditions such as chronic venous insufficiency, venous ulcers, and deep vein thrombosis. Understanding these complications highlights the importance of early diagnosis and appropriate management.

CHRONIC VENOUS INSUFFICIENCY (CVI)

Definition and Pathophysiology:

Chronic Venous Insufficiency (CVI) occurs when the venous wall and/or valves in the leg veins are not working effectively, making it difficult for blood to return to the heart from the legs. CVI leads to increased blood pressure in the veins which can cause further valve damage and venous reflux (blood flowing backward).

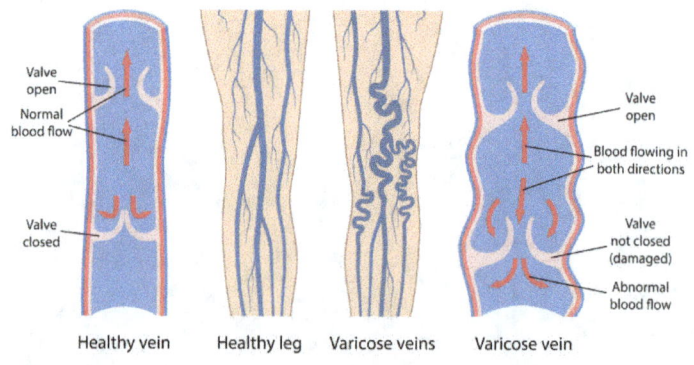

Symptoms
- Swelling in the legs and ankles, especially after extended periods of standing.
- A feeling of heaviness or cramps in the legs.
- Pain that improves when legs are raised.
- Changes in skin color, especially around the ankles.
- Varicose veins are often present.

Management
Treatment focuses on alleviating symptoms and stopping further progression. Strategies include:
- Compression stockings to aid blood flow.
- Exercise programs to improve venous pump function.
- Procedures such as sclerotherapy, laser therapy, or vein stripping might be necessary in advanced cases.

Venous Ulcers

Definition and Development

Venous ulcers are open sores that occur when the increased pressure in the veins of the lower leg causes fluid to leak into surrounding tissues, resulting in swelling, tissue breakdown, and eventually ulceration. They typically appear near the ankle and can be slow to heal.

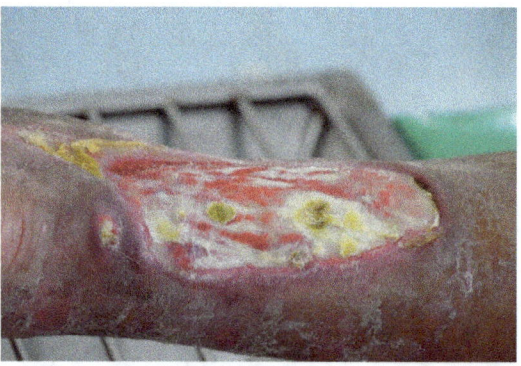

Symptoms
- New or worsening pain around the affected area.

- Swelling, itching, and redness around the ulcer.
- Discharge from the ulcer.
- Skin discoloration and hardening around the ulcer.

Management

Effective management of venous ulcers involves:

- Compression therapy to reduce edema and enhance circulation.
- Regular wound care, including cleaning and dressing the ulcer.
- Keeping the affected leg elevated when possible.
- In severe cases, skin grafting or other surgical interventions may be necessary.

DEEP VEIN THROMBOSIS (DVT)

Definition and Risk Factors

DVT is a condition in which a blood clot forms in a deep vein, typically in the legs. Risk factors include prolonged immobility, certain medical conditions that affect blood clotting, surgery, and trauma. People with varicosity are at an increased risk due to altered blood flow and vein damage.

Symptoms

- Swelling in one or both legs.
- Pain or tenderness in the leg, which may only be present when standing or walking.
- Warmth and redness in the affected area.

Management

DVT is a medical emergency due to the risk of the clot dislodging and traveling to the lungs, causing a potentially fatal pulmonary embolism.

- Anticoagulant medications are the primary treatment to prevent further clotting.
- Compression stockings and elevation of the affected leg can help relieve symptoms.
- In severe cases, thrombolytic therapy to dissolve the clot or surgical intervention may be necessary.

GLOSSARY OF TERMS

Anticoagulant

A type of medication that helps prevent blood clots from forming by reducing the blood's ability to coagulate. Anticoagulants are commonly used to treat and prevent conditions such as deep vein thrombosis (DVT) and pulmonary embolism.

Arteries

Blood vessels that carry oxygenated blood away from the heart to the rest of the body. Arteries have thick, elastic walls that withstand high pressure exerted by the heart's pumping action.

Capillaries

The smallest blood vessels in the body, capillaries connect arteries to veins and facilitate the exchange of oxygen, carbon dioxide, nutrients, and waste products between blood and tissues.

Chronic Venous Insufficiency (CVI)

A condition that occurs when the leg veins are not able to pump enough blood back to the heart due to damaged valves or blocked veins, leading to blood pooling and increased pressure in the veins, which can cause varicose veins and other symptoms.

Compression Therapy

A treatment method involving the use of specially designed stockings or bandages that apply gentle pressure to the legs. This therapy helps improve blood flow and reduce swelling and is commonly used to manage symptoms of varicose veins and venous insufficiency.

Deep Vein Thrombosis (DVT)

A medical condition where a blood clot forms in a deep vein, usually in the legs. DVT can cause pain and swelling and may lead to serious complications if the clot travels to the lungs, causing a pulmonary embolism.

Doppler Ultrasound

A non-invasive imaging technique that uses high-frequency sound waves to measure the flow of blood through the veins and arteries. This method is widely used to diagnose conditions such as varicose veins, venous insufficiency, and blood flow blockages.

Edema

Swelling caused by excess fluid trapped in the body's tissues. Edema commonly affects the legs, ankles, and feet and can be a symptom of various health issues, including venous insufficiency, heart failure, and kidney disease.

Endovascular

A term referring to procedures that are performed within the blood vessels through small incisions, using catheters and other minimally invasive techniques. Endovascular procedures are used to diagnose and treat vascular conditions without the need for open surgery.

Endovenous Laser Treatment (EVLT)

A minimally invasive laser treatment used to close off varicose veins. A laser fiber is inserted into the vein, and laser energy is applied to heat and collapse the vein, rerouting blood flow to healthier veins.

Flavonoids

A group of natural substances found in fruits, vegetables, grains, bark, roots, stems, flowers, tea, and wine. Flavonoids are known for their antioxidant properties and are believed to enhance vascular health by strengthening capillaries and reducing inflammation.

Foam Sclerotherapy

A form of sclerotherapy that involves injecting a foam solution into the vein, causing it to scar and close. This technique is particularly effective for larger varicose veins and helps redirect blood to healthier veins.

Genetics

Refers to the study of genes and their roles in inheritance. In the context of varicosity, genetics can determine an individual's predisposition to developing varicose veins, as certain genetic factors may influence the strength and functionality of venous walls and valves.

Hemorrhoids

Swollen veins in the lowest part of the rectum and anus that, similar to varicose veins, can become painful and may bleed. Hemorrhoids can be caused by increased pressure during bowel movements, pregnancy, or due to chronic constipation.

Hormonal Changes

Alterations in the body's hormone levels, which can affect the tone and elasticity of venous walls. Hormonal changes are significant during pregnancy, menopause, or as a result of using hormonal medications, impacting the development of varicosities.

Intermittent Pneumatic Compression Devices

Medical devices used to help improve venous circulation in the limbs by mechanically inflating and deflating air-filled cuffs around the legs. These devices mimic the natural pumping action of muscles to help prevent blood clots and manage symptoms of venous insufficiency.

Leg Ulcers

Open sores or wounds on the legs that do not heal normally and are often caused by poor blood circulation due to venous insufficiency. These ulcers can become chronic and are susceptible to infection and further complications.

Lipodermatosclerosis

A chronic skin and tissue condition often associated with severe chronic venous insufficiency, characterized by thickening and hardening of the skin on the lower legs, making it appear tapered like an inverted bottle.

Magnetic Resonance (MR) Venography

A non-invasive imaging test that uses magnetic resonance technology to visualize veins throughout the body. MR venography is used for diagnosing venous diseases including deep vein thrombosis and assessing the veins in patients with varicose veins.

Mechanochemical Ablation (MOCA)

A minimally invasive treatment for varicose veins that combines mechanical disruption of the vein with a chemical sclerosant to close the affected veins without the use of heat.

Micronized Purified Flavonoid Fraction (MPFF)

A venoactive drug made from flavonoids, primarily used to treat venous circulation disorders. MPFF is known to reduce inflammation, protect the vascular structure, and improve venous tone.

Obesity

A condition characterized by excess body fat, which increases the risk of developing varicose veins due to higher pressure exerted on the venous system, impairing blood flow and contributing to venous insufficiency.

Pelvic Congestion Syndrome (PCS)

A chronic condition that occurs when varicose veins form in the pelvic area, often causing chronic pelvic pain. The condition is predominantly found in women and can be related to hormonal changes and venous insufficiency.

Phlebitis

Inflammation of a vein, usually in the legs, which can occur in both superficial and deep veins. Phlebitis can cause redness, swelling, and pain, and may lead to more serious complications if not treated properly.

Photoplethysmography

A non-invasive optical technique used to detect blood volume changes in the microvascular bed of tissue. It is often used in the diagnosis and monitoring of peripheral arterial and venous diseases.

Plethysmography

A diagnostic procedure used to measure changes in volume within an organ or body part through various methods, often used to assess the amount of blood in the legs to help diagnose conditions such as deep vein thrombosis.

Post-thrombotic Syndrome (PTS)

A long-term complication that can occur following a deep vein thrombosis (DVT), characterized by chronic pain, swelling, and skin changes in the affected limb, and sometimes venous ulcers.

Pulmonary Circulation

The segment of the circulatory system which carries deoxygenated blood from the right side of the heart to the lungs to become oxygenated and then back to the left side of the heart to be pumped to the rest of the body.

Pulmonary Embolism

A potentially life-threatening complication, often occurring when a blood clot from a deep vein (like those from the legs) travels to the lungs, blocking one or more arteries. Prompt treatment is critical to prevent severe consequences or death.

Radiofrequency Ablation (RFA)

A minimally invasive treatment that uses radiofrequency energy to heat and collapse diseased varicose veins, sealing them off and rerouting blood to healthier veins.

Reticular Varicosities

A type of varicose vein that forms a network of blue or green veins, typically smaller than trunk varicose veins but larger than spider veins, often located just beneath the skin's surface.

Saphenous Vein

A large vein extending from the ankle to the groin, divided into the great and small saphenous veins, commonly involved in varicose vein procedures due to its length and surface location.

Sclerotherapy

A treatment for varicose and spider veins where a solution is injected into the vein, causing it to scar and blood to reroute through healthier veins, eventually leading the treated vein to collapse and fade.

Skin Pigmentation

Changes in skin color that can occur around varicose veins due to the leakage of blood or iron from the veins into the surrounding tissues, often resulting in a brownish discoloration.

Spider Veins

Small, damaged veins that can appear on the surface of the legs or face and are smaller than varicose veins; they are often red, blue, or purple and look like thin lines, webs, or branches.

Superficial Thrombophlebitis

An inflammatory condition due to a blood clot in a superficial vein, characterized by redness, warmth, and pain along the affected vein, commonly occurring in the legs.

Systemic Circulation

The part of the cardiovascular system which carries oxygenated blood away from the heart to the body, and returns deoxygenated blood back to the heart.

Telangiectasias

Also known as spider veins, these are small, broken or widened blood vessels that appear near the surface of the skin, often red or blue in color.

Thermablation

A group of minimally invasive procedures that use heat to treat varicose veins, including techniques like endovenous laser therapy and radiofrequency ablation.

Trendelenburg Test

A diagnostic test used to assess the competence of the venous valves in the superficial and deep venous systems of the legs, involving leg elevation and tourniquet application.

Tunica Adventitia

The outermost layer of a blood vessel composed of connective tissue that provides structural support and flexibility to the vessel.

Tunica Intima

The innermost layer of a blood vessel that includes a lining of endothelial cells that provides a smooth surface for blood to flow over and contains the valves in veins.

Tunica Media

The middle layer of a blood vessel made up of smooth muscle and elastic fibers, allowing the vessel to regulate its diameter under the influence of the autonomic nervous system.

Ultrasound

A diagnostic imaging technique that uses high-frequency sound waves to create images of structures within the body, commonly used to evaluate the condition of veins and arteries.

Valves

Structures within veins that maintain blood flow in one direction back towards the heart, preventing backflow and pooling of blood.

Varicoceles

Enlargements of the veins within the scrotum, akin to varicose veins, which can cause pain and reproductive issues.

Varicose Veins

Enlarged, swollen, and twisting veins, often appearing blue or dark purple, caused by faulty valves within the veins that allow blood to pool rather than flow efficiently.

Varicosity

The condition characterized by enlarged, dilated veins due to valve insufficiencies, commonly manifesting as varicose veins.

Veins

Blood vessels that carry blood toward the heart, equipped with valves that help prevent the backflow of blood.

Venography

An imaging test that involves injecting contrast dye into the veins to visualize them during an X-ray, used to diagnose conditions like deep vein thrombosis.

Venous Circulation

The part of the circulatory system that returns deoxygenated blood back to the heart, involving all veins and venous blood vessels.

Venous Insufficiency

A condition where the flow of blood through the veins is inadequate, causing blood to pool in the veins, often leading to varicose veins and other complications.

Venous Valves

Small structures within veins that open and close to control blood flow toward the heart, preventing backflow and ensuring efficient venous return.

Afterword

As we close the pages of "The Varicosity Handbook," it is my hope that this guide has not only enlightened you about varicosity but also empowered you with the knowledge to navigate this common but often misunderstood condition. Varicose veins touch the lives of millions around the globe, transcending boundaries of age, gender, and lifestyle, making it imperative that we deepen our understanding and enhance our approach to dealing with this ailment.

Throughout this book, we have journeyed through the intricacies of the circulatory system, explored the underlying mechanisms of varicosity, and discussed the various manifestations and complications associated with this condition. Each chapter was crafted to provide you with a comprehensive view, from basic definitions to advanced treatment options, ensuring a well-rounded grasp of both the concept and the clinical aspects of varicose veins.

The management of varicosity is multifaceted, involving lifestyle changes, medical interventions, and sometimes surgical procedures. It has been my aim to present these topics in a manner that is both accessible and practical, providing actionable advice for those affected and their caregivers.

The discussions on innovative treatments and ongoing research underscore the dynamic nature of vascular medicine and the continuous efforts to improve patient outcomes.

I would like to extend my heartfelt thanks to the many patients, colleagues, and medical professionals who have shared their experiences and insights, enriching the content of this book. Their contributions have been invaluable in portraying the real-world implications of varicosity and the human element underlying the medical descriptions.

As varicosity management continues to evolve, I encourage you to stay informed and proactive. Engage with healthcare providers, participate in support groups, and advocate for your health. Remember, the journey to better vascular health is ongoing, and with the right knowledge and resources, you can lead a healthier, more comfortable life.

Lastly, whether you are a patient, a medical student, or a practitioner, I hope this handbook serves as a useful resource for years to come. Together, let us continue to advance our understanding and treatment of varicosity, striving for excellence in care and improvements in quality of life.

Thank you for joining me in exploring the fascinating world of varicosity. May this book inspire you to learn more, ask questions, and seek the best possible care.

Mohammad E. Barbati

ABOUT THE AUTHOR

Dr. Mohammad E. Barbati is a consultant vascular and endovascular surgeon. He obtained an MD in endovascular treatment of venous diseases from University Hospital, Aachen. In 2018 he was appointed as a consultant vascular surgeon and lecturer at University Hospital Aachen. Dr. Barbati has been a principal or co-investigator in several clinical trials and studies involving 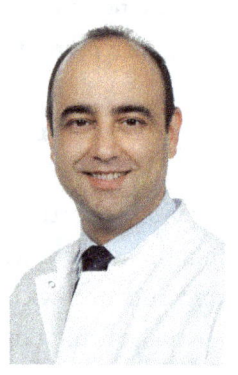 interventional treatment of DVT, PCS, PTS and other vascular diseases. To date, he has authored or co-authored more than 60 scientific publications, abstracts and book chapters. He has given over 100 invited lectures at national and international meetings and is a consultant to many medical device manufacturers.

www.ingramcontent.com/pod-product-compliance
Lightning Source LLC
Chambersburg PA
CBHW071508220526
45472CB00003B/956